Alison's Story

MARY & ANDREW PEACH

Published by YPS

A CIP catalogue record for this book is available from the British Library.

ISBN 978-1-84263-155-3

Book layout and cover design by Clare Brayshaw

Prepared and printed by:

York Publishing Services Ltd
64 Hallfield Road
Layerthorpe
York YO31 7ZQ

Tel: 01904 431213

Website: www.yps-publishing.co.uk

This story is dedicated to Giles and Thomas,
Alison's brothers, whom she dearly loved
and who enriched her life.

Introduction

Talking to friends over the last few weeks, we have been surprised by the number of people telling us how much Alison had influenced their lives. We too have begun to realise what a remarkable person she was and what a hard act she is to follow.

Alison ignored her handicap and got on with life as if her condition was quite normal.

She saw everyone as a friend and greeted them accordingly.

She was kind to people before they were kind to her.

She accepted everyone for who they were.

She didn't have an evil thought about anybody, not even in the deepest recesses of her mind.

She never complained about anything or anyone.

Every morning, when Alison woke, she got up straightaway and was ready and keen to start a new day.

She was enthusiastic about everything.

She was a mature person who showed enormous courage in facing life with a very visible handicap.

It is with these thoughts in mind that we have decided to write a short account entitled 'Alison's Story', so that future generations will know what a special person she was and how privileged we are to have been her family.

Chapter 1

Birth and Early Years

Alison, our first child, was born at 9 Victoria Way, Outwood, Wakefield, in the early hours of Wednesday 2nd November 1966. Later that day the doctor called to examine her, and he asked Andrew to go to his surgery to pick up some eye drops. Once there, he told Andrew that Alison had been born with Down's syndrome and that Mary was not to be told.

After a few days the doctor made another visit and said that he might have been mistaken, and perhaps it was just the old Peach face, but he still wasn't sure. A week later, he called again and this time said he now thought Alison had Down's syndrome but could not be absolutely certain. He said he would leave it a bit longer to see how she developed, but he still did not want anything said to Mary. After a further six weeks he called again and confirmed his suspicion, but said Alison would need to see a specialist and would probably need a blood test as final confirmation. He also made it clear that Mary should still not be told and that he would tell her at the appropriate time.

Christmas came and went with the customary celebrations and festivities. The following February we arranged a short holiday in a cottage in Ambleside. Mary's sister Chris, her husband Gerry, and their five-year-old twin boys, Nick and Chris, came too. It was cold in the Lake District and, despite a smoky fire in the living room keeping us warm, Alison developed a rash round her neck which was severe enough for us to take her to see the local doctor. Andrew was terrified that the doctor would comment on Alison's disability, but he said nothing and prescribed some cream that relieved our concern and eventually saw off the rash. We didn't know until years later that, shortly after Alison's birth, Chris had met the midwife crying on the stairs at our home and that she had told Chris about Alison's condition!

Back from the holiday, life went on much as you would expect with a young baby in the house. After Alison was born we had a lot of difficulty getting her to take food, but by this time she was eating well and was starting to enjoy a good bowl of Farlene. She was now sitting up unaided and had developed a natty trick of moving her legs from in front of her to behind her without moving her trunk: as if her hips were double-jointed.

In those days, each mum with a new-born child was allocated a health visitor, who called from time to time to check that the baby was developing properly. On one of these visits, when Alison was about six months old, Mary mentioned this 'trick' to the health visitor who, without any preamble, immediately said, "Well you know she's not normal. She is a mongol and will never grow up. She won't walk or talk and her hair won't grow. You don't have to look after her. I can take her now if you want me to. Anyway, I'll have to go."

It is impossible to imagine how distraught Mary must have felt. She was very distressed and rang Andrew at work. He came home straightaway and explained, as best he could, the uncertainty there had been over Alison's condition and the insistence of the doctor that he would tell her at the appropriate time. When Mary told Andrew about the health visitor suggesting that Alison could be taken from them, they both knew, there and then, that they would love Alison with all their hearts and take care of her no matter what the future held. Chris arrived promptly to give support, and has been the main family support ever since.

A day or so later, we saw the doctor to arrange blood tests for the three of us. At the hospital in Leeds where the tests were carried out, the consultant took Alison off to see two other specialists. Of the three of them, two were of the opinion that Alison had Down's syndrome and the other thought it was highly likely. A week or so later, having received the test results, the doctor confirmed that Alison had, indeed, Down's syndrome. He also said that we were not at any particular risk of having another Down's baby, and he encouraged us to have more children.

One evening, just after this period, Alison was lying quietly in her pram with a pull-string doll dangling from the hood when, suddenly and unexpectedly, we heard the characteristic clack-clack which these dolls make when the string is pulled. We both rushed over to the pram to find that Alison had stretched up, taken hold of the string, and given it a good tug. We will never forget the delight, even excitement, this gave us as we realised that Alison had the ability to work out simple things for herself. Although this was a small event, in our minds it was hugely significant, and it gave us great hope and encouragement. It is ironic that all of the experts portrayed Alison as a burden we would have to manage (apart from the health visitor who offered to take her off our hands), but it was Alison herself who gave us hope for the future and a taste of what was to come.

In June that year, we had a holiday with Andrew's parents in a hotel at Mudeford in Dorset. The hotel had an outdoor pool where Alison had her first experience of splashing about. She clearly enjoyed it, and perhaps it set the scene for her future main sporting activity, swimming. That August, in France, she had her first experience of camping: sleeping in a tiny tent with the ridge pole missing and Mum cooking on a primus stove.

In February, 1968, we moved to a much bigger house at 421 Barnsley Road, Wakefield. At the time, Mary was pregnant with Giles who was expected in May. Alison was now 16 months old. Although not yet walking unaided, she had learned to use her sit-in baby walker with considerable dexterity; carrying it most of the time, and just using it to sit down when she reached her destination. She was also developing her vocabulary. She was able to say 'mum-mum' and 'da-da', and 'yes' and 'no' (mainly 'no'); was able to ask for a drink by saying 'ki-ki'; and was eating and sleeping well; although she invariably woke in the middle of the night for a 'ki-ki'. The Barnsley Road house was on the A61 trunk road: a very busy route into town used by many of our friends. We constantly had visitors, particularly on Saturdays. This became part of normal life, and we received many invitations to visit friends' homes in return. Our friends always made a fuss of Alison and she would smile and beam when spoken to.

Giles was born at home at about 10 a.m. on Saturday 25th May. It was a beautiful day. As the midwife was helping with the delivery, we could hear Alison rattling around in her baby walker on the parquet floor in the hall. The birth went without a hitch and all our Saturday morning friends started turning up as usual for coffee. They were completely unaware of what had just transpired. According to the disapproving midwife, we had over twenty visitors before lunch.

In July that year, we went on holiday to Mablethorpe, where we stayed in a chalet near the beach. We were delighted to have Chris, Gerry and Nick and Chris, to stay for a few days. It was during this stay that, with the help of the twins steadying her, one on each side, Alison finally walked unaided. We were frightened to let her go to sleep in case she had forgotten how to walk when she woke up. However, the next day all was well and she literally never looked back.

Back home, life went on as usual and we spent a happy Christmas enjoying the excitement and drama of the first manned mission to the moon. Alison got a rocking horse from Father Christmas: the type that you sit in, with a strong chair as a seat instead of a saddle. She soon got the knack of moving backwards and forwards to get it rocking; eventually with such vigour that the animal used to work its way across the floor. It was at Barnsley Road that she started to entertain us with some unexpected skills: the first time she unzipped a banana without Mary's help, she bit the end off and stood it straight up on the bitten end; she used to do the splits quite easily, which she later, for some unexplained reason, referred to as 'doing the blisters'; her feet were unusually flexible, and she would pick up toys with her toes as a matter of routine. Once, when on a picnic and sitting on a rug, she used her big and next toe to pick up a spoon and load it with baked beans!

Earlier, in October 1968, Andrew gained his final qualification in civil engineering, and we decided it was time for a change, so he started looking for another job. The search took some time to come to fruition. During this period Alison continued to develop, to all intents and purposes, normally. We had a nice holiday in May 1969. Chris and Gerry had by this time moved to Stourbridge, and we stayed in their house whilst they were away on their holidays. In the summer, we moved to Dundee and Andrew started work in the City Engineer's Department.

Our house in Wakefield took some time to sell so, after a week staying in a caravan at Coupar Angus, we moved into a council flat. It was on the fifth floor of a tower block at Ardler, which was just off the city ring road (a development since demolished). Despite having little stimulation outside the flat, Alison continued to thrive. Mary spent a lot of time playing with her and Giles and took them out whenever the weather permitted. Alison quickly became a favourite of the elderly lady in the flat next door.

Finally, our house in Wakefield was sold. In January 1970 we moved to our new permanent home. This was a small bungalow at 45 Torridon Road, Broughty Ferry. Broughty Ferry is a pretty, former fishing village which by then was a suburb to the east of Dundee. Straightaway, we were welcomed by our new neighbours who were all of a similar age to us and had young families. Alison easily took to her new set of friends, both children and parents. They, in turn, took to her and had a big impact on her early development. Soon after we arrived, Alison went off exploring the new neighbourhood on her own. She managed to get herself shut in the porch of one of the bungalows across the road. Mary noticed that she had gone missing and soon located her, only to find that the porch door was now locked and the occupants were out. In a panic, Mary climbed into the house through an open window. She had just opened the front door when the owners of the house returned home. After the initial surprise, it was laughter all round. We still meet this couple regularly, even after all these years.

The same lady had a friend who taught at the Demonstration School in Dundee. This was a primary school attached to the Dundee Teacher Training College. We will always be grateful to this neighbour and her friend for arranging for Alison to attend the school when she was still only three years old. She was the only pupil with special needs. However, no concessions were made to her handicap and she was treated in exactly the same way as all the other children. She was very happy there and frequently came home covered in poster paint. After Alison had passed away, her teacher contacted us and wrote, "I fondly remember how Alison diligently tackled an inset puzzle of a tipper truck offloading red apples. She tipped out the puzzle every day and, piece by piece, she worked out how to complete it herself, without any help. Alison loved painting at the easel and enjoyed helping to wash it down at tidy-up time". Her teacher went on to write, "Music was another great interest, and she always responded with great enthusiasm". During this period, using flash cards, Mary had made good progress in getting Alison to read. She attached the appropriate words to pieces of furniture, kitchen equipment and other household items. However, enrolling at the Demonstration School was one of the most important and beneficial events for her future development. We were indeed blessed with good friends in Scotland.

We spent two years living in Broughty Ferry, during which time Giles learnt to walk, talk, run errands for his mum and play out with his friends. He seemed instinctively to know that Alison was special, but he still competed with her for toys and attention, as siblings do. This 'competition' spurred Alison on. Her vocabulary came on in leaps and bounds, and she quickly learned to read the TV schedules to make sure she didn't miss anything she wanted to watch. On summer days, Mary and a neighbour would fill our VW Beetle with excited young children and take them to the beach. Alison was always in the thick of these adventures. As one of the gang, she joined in all the fun with her usual enthusiasm.

We had two annual holidays during our time in Scotland. The first, in June 1970, was a camping holiday on the west coast. We arrived at our first site in pouring rain. Undaunted, we donned our oilskins and hired a rowing boat on an adjacent loch. Alison had always been uncannily sensitive to potential danger. She would signal her concerns by saying "No like it", to which our usual reply was "No choice!", and we would carry on with what we were doing. On this occasion, fear obviously got hold of her in a big way. As she was lifted into the boat she shouted "No like it" then, recognising the inevitable, completed the sentence by adding "No choice!". After that "No like it. No choice" became part of the family vocabulary. In October the following year we went on a package holiday to Malgrat de Mar in Spain. It was Alison's first experience of flying and she managed without any problem, unlike in later years, when flying became a major fear for her.

By the end of 1971, for family reasons, we decided to move to Hull where Andrew would join the family engineering business. At the very start of 1972, after another unforgettable Hogmanay, we took up temporary residence in Andrew's father's house in Kirk Ella.

This move produced an immediate problem: Alison was now five years old and had had almost two years of schooling in Dundee, but the East Riding did not school special needs children until they were seven. In order to try and overcome this problem, Mary managed to get a meeting with the Council's educational psychologist. We took Alison with us to meet the him. After a brief discussion and a few simple tests, he said that he didn't see any reason why Alison shouldn't go to a normal school and he arranged for her to attend St. Andrew's Primary School in Kirk Ella. She was the first Down's child to be placed in a mainstream school in the East Riding: she had no additional support.

In May we moved to our new permanent home at 9 Annandale Road, Kirk Ella. Alison, again, quickly made friends with other children in the road and would call on them if no-one was out playing. In a way, life picked up in Kirk Ella where it had left off in Dundee. A neighbour, Carol, who lived just up the road with her husband, a heart specialist from the Middle East, and their two children,

Karrime and Nassime told us that one day Alison had knocked at their door and asked if Hassam and Kassam were coming out to play! Alison was happy at school, and made friends with both children and parents. One of the parents, Ken Knighton, was Hull City's star football player. Alison would leave Mary and grasp Ken's free hand as he took his own child into school. When she came out, she would run straight to him. He would lift her onto his shoulders and carry her to Mary waiting at the gate.

Thomas was born in the Westwood Maternity Hospital in Beverley on 1st August 1972. When Mary was in hospital having Thomas, Alison decided that she had some important duties to undertake as Mum's deputy. These included polishing the furniture, which she did with Germolene ointment: the house smelt nice and clean when Mary and Thomas came home!

Every Saturday, when Thomas was still a baby, Grandpa (Andrew's father) took Alison and Giles to a hotel for lunch. They looked forward to this, as a special treat. They often spoke about it in later years, particularly when we drove past the hotel.

In May 1973, we again embarked on a package holiday, this time to Lloret de Mar. We stayed in a multi-storey hotel and had two adjacent rooms on the 5th floor: Mum, Dad and Thomas in one room, Alison and Giles in the other. With three children, it was quite an active holiday. We took to having a rest on the balcony after lunch, whilst the children played in the room with various toys. One day Alison slipped out unnoticed, after having first locked us on the balcony. To rub salt into the wound, when we looked over the handrail we could see her playing by the pool. Andrew had a bit of a nervy climb from one balcony to the next, before being able to get back into the appropriate room and rescue Mary.

That summer, just before the start of the school holidays, we had an unexpected visit from two of Alison's teachers. They came to warn us that the headmistress at St. Andrew's wanted Alison out of the school. Apparently, Alison used to get bored in the singing classes (which the headmistress took) and used to undo other children's ribbons and shoelaces. The teachers told us that they were not surprised she got bored, and affirmed that she was quite capable of staying at the school for the time being. Alison had clearly won the teachers' hearts, but had not endeared herself to the headmistress. We were not happy with her attending a school where she was not wanted, so she transferred to Hessle School. This school was housed in a large, relatively new building, with an annexe for special needs pupils. The annexe was situated in the old school building at the other side of the playing field. The staff were marvellous – some of their names became legendary in our family – and Alison was very happy there. At a parents' evening one of her classmates told us that, when the teacher left the classroom, Alison went to the front and took over. We are still in touch with parents from that time, and occasionally see a couple of the pupils who are now nearing middle age.

In the first few years after leaving Scotland, when the children were still quite young, we made several visits to stay with our former neighbours. When Alison first saw our old house, she opened the gate and ran down the path shouting, "I've found it! I've found it!". She then embraced the front door, which had recently been painted, and was still tacky. On another occasion, in late autumn, we visited a beach in Fife. It was a windy, rainy day and the sea was quite rough. On the beach a pole, a bit like a short telegraph pole, was sticking vertically out of the sand to a height of about six feet. As the waves came in the pole was covered to a depth of about two feet, and as the waves went out they just passed the foot of the pole, leaving it clear of water for a few seconds. Giles and his friend, Keith, started to play at running down the beach, briefly hugging the pole, and retreating just before a wave returned. Alison watched this with interest and then decided to have a go herself. Unfortunately, she got the timing totally out of sync, and arrived at the pole in time to hug it just as the water came up above her waist. She came back looking quite triumphant, although a little puzzled.

On another occasion we went go-karting. It was a fairly short track with rather slow karts: fast enough to attract adults but slow enough for older children to have a go. Alison watched Giles and other children go on the karts and decided she would like a turn. She donned the crash helmet, which was far too large, and sat down in the driver's seat. We were slightly alarmed and felt that she might need some help, so Andrew managed to crouch just behind her, on a tiny bit of engine mounting, with his bottom right over the nearside back wheel. The 'man' said to Alison, "That's the accelerator", upon which she pressed firmly on the pedal and the kart took off at full speed in a straight line. It went off the track, scattering the safety tyres, over a grass mound, down the other side, and across the track again, scattering a few more tyres. Fortunately, at this point Andrew managed to kick Alison's foot off the accelerator and the kart came to a sudden stop.

For over forty years, as a child and an adult, Alison had many happy visits to Scotland and was always warmly welcomed by our Scottish friends.

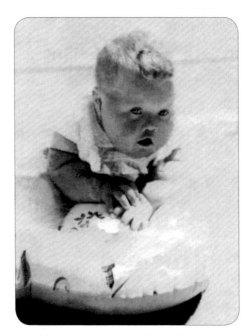

First Holiday – Mudeford 1967

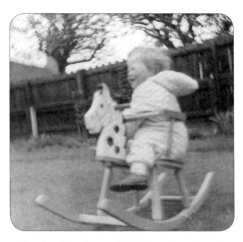

In the Garden – 421 Barnsley Road

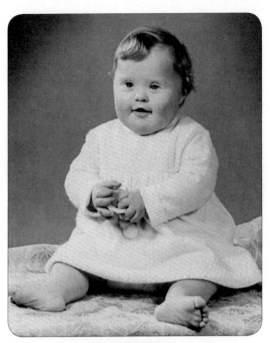

First Birthday

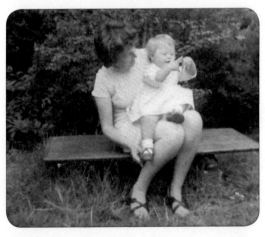

With Aunty Chris doing Incy-wincy Spider

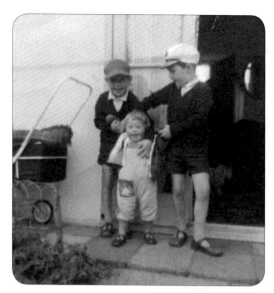

With Nick & Chris at Mablethorpe – 1968

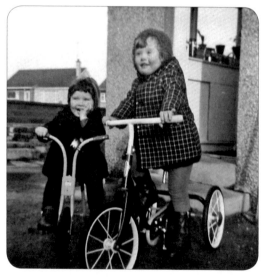

45 Torridon Road, Broughty Ferry – 1970

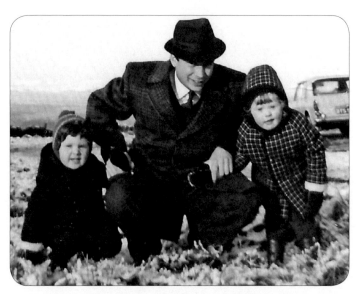

Scotland in Winter – 1970/71

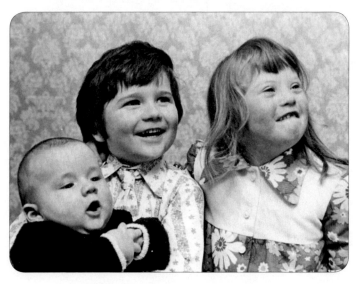

With Thomas and Giles – 1972

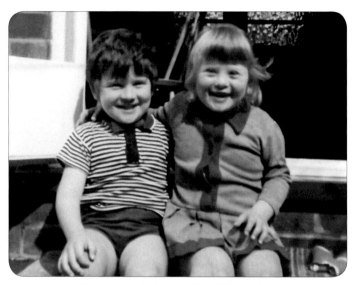

9 Annandale Road, Kirk Ella – 1972

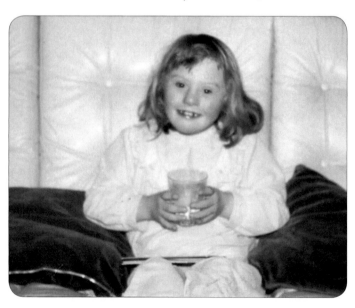

At Aunty Chris's in Stourbridge

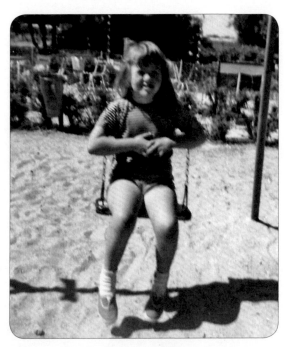

Pornic – 1976

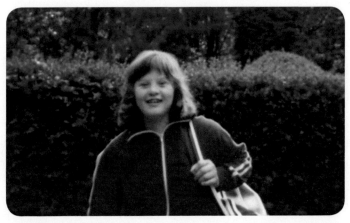

238 West Ella Road – 1st Day at Etton Pasture School 1977

Chapter 2

Alison in West Ella

In April 1977 we moved to our present house, 238 West Ella Road, West Ella. It is a semi-detached house with a large garden. Since she was quite small, Alison had spent many happy hours playing with her toy pram and dolls. She used to talk to the dolls, dressing and undressing them and putting them in the pram, just as you would have expected any little girl to do. By the time we moved to West Ella, she was also playing more imaginative games with some of her brothers' toys. On one occasion, she put on a toy storm trooper's helmet, picked up a toy rifle, pointed it at her Dad, and shouted, "Hands Up!". Andrew was sitting reading a newspaper at the time and didn't take much notice. Suddenly, the rifle barrel came straight through the paper and dug him hard in the ribs. With a cry of pain, Andrew dropped the paper and put his hands up to avoid further punishment, which he was certain would follow.

When we moved to West Ella we became regular attenders at the Methodist Church in the village. Alison knew everyone in the small congregation as well as all the local preachers. A member of the church confessed to Mary that she could not take her eyes off Alison. She was astonished to see Alison open her hymn book at the right page and lustily sing all the words. More recently, another member recalls wondering why her children were once having hysterics during a carol service. It turned out that Alison, who was in the pew behind them, had sung "While shepherds washed their socks at night" instead of "While shepherds watched their flocks by night". Alison occasionally read a short lesson and once played her keyboard, although she got rather cross with herself when she played a wrong note. She was good at 'asides' (personal comments not meant for general hearing), but she tended to say them in a stage whisper. One of Alison's 'asides' occurred as the Minister at that time, Rev. Geoff Dougal, entered the church from the vestry to take the service. A loud "Geoff's had his hair cut" was received with gales of laughter by the assembled worshippers. Geoff had clearly had a rather severe short back and sides. Alison firmly believed in the Bible and was in demand whenever there was a quiz at the Church Youth Club – where she also acted as the DJ. She used to go roller-skating with the Youth Club. She didn't actually put any skates on, but still got onto the rink and moved around, sliding her feet backwards and forwards with all the others in a pretty good simulation of a competent skater. On another occasion, when the radio was on in the house, she heard Gerald Priestland, the BBC Religious Affairs reporter, introduce a programme by asking the question, "Who was Jesus Christ?". Alison replied with some disdain, "Everyone knows that! It was Robert Powell". Robert Powell was the actor who had taken the part of Jesus in a recently released film. Alison was also good at general TV quizzes and made uncannily correct choices from multiple choice questions. She shouted her answers at the screen, as if the contestants could hear her!

She got to know one family in the village, Hazel, John and their two daughters, particularly well. They had an early introduction to Alison's character when they gave her a lift in their car. Alison took the front seat, as was her custom, and proceeded to open the electric sun-roof. Hazel was driving and the two girls were seated in the back. The girls immediately complained that it was cold, to which Alison replied firmly, "It'll do you good". That was the end of that conversation. John often picked Alison up from CASE when we were not available. He had a painting and decorating business and used to collect Alison in his van. He recalls how she loved to climb up into the cab from where she had an excellent view of all that was going on. She would entertain John with pertinent comments about anything and everything she saw. After she had passed away, John used his considerable artistic talents to produce a lovely portrait of Alison which captures perfectly her happy, smiling nature. We have it hanging on the wall for all to see and to remember Alison, just as she was.

In the summer of the year we went to live in West Ella, Alison, who was now eleven, left the school at Hessle and moved to Etton Pasture Special School. This was housed in a single storey, post-war, prefabricated building set in fields on the outskirts of Etton, a village about five miles from Beverley (the building was demolished in 2011). Alison used to be collected from the house each day by a yellow school bus and dropped off again in the late afternoon. The journey could take up to an hour and a half and the children were accompanied by a supervisor who kept order by discouraging conversation. Alison went down almost every road in the East Riding. We realised this because, when we went out in the car and passed the end of a street, she told us who lived there. She was always keen to go for a ride in the car, taking a lively interest in anything unusual. Once she saw a hawk flapping its wings and hovering over a hedgerow, looking for prey: she informed us that the bird was 'stuck'. On another occasion, when at the wheel, Andrew took a quick swig from a can of Coke: she rebuked him with, "Dad, don't drink and drive!".

Etton Pastures, as the school was widely known, was run by Geoff Pyatt and his wife, Gwyneth. She had fiery red hair and was equally fiery in her teaching approach. At a parents' evening, she told us of an early encounter she had had with Alison. Apparently, Alison had been sitting in a classroom next to her friend, Linda, when Gwyneth went in. Alison immediately dug an elbow into Linda's ribs and, looking straight at Gwyneth, said, "We don't like her, do we, Linda?". We went to every parents' evening and always got a good report. At one of these evenings, the teacher informed us, to our surprise, that she had seen our wedding photos. Alison must have sneaked them out of the house in her school bag and put them back when she got home.

The headmaster at Etton Pastures did not like any pupil sitting at a desk after their fourteenth birthday. Therefore Alison spent her last two years doing art, crafts, gardening and working in the kitchen. It was at Etton, in the spring of 1982, that Alison gained her Duke of Edinburgh's Bronze Award. This required her to pass tests in everything from cookery to map reading, and included a twelve mile hike in the Yorkshire Wolds. Notwithstanding Gwyneth being 'around', Alison had a very happy five years at the school, and often recalled many of the teachers by name, always referring to them with great affection. A year or so before the school was demolished, we drove out, at her request, to see it. It looked very sad and derelict. She was keen to go inside, which we did. As she took photographs, she explained who had taught in each, by then hardly recognisable, classroom.

When she was coming to the end of her final year at Etton, we and other parents asked the school what the future options were for our young people. The school arranged for us to be addressed by representatives from the Council's Education Department, but we were told that we would not be allowed to ask questions. Very little was learnt from the meeting, and it quickly became apparent that nothing concrete was in place. We were left wondering why no post-sixteen courses were available for pupils with special needs.

One of the parents, Martin, contacted Hull College of Further Education to see if they could help. The upshot was a meeting with the Principal. He was very sympathetic and arranged for a two-year course to be set up specifically for people with learning disabilities. At the time, the College had an empty building on Charterhouse Lane, close to its main campus. The building was referred to as the Charterhouse Annexe and that was where the course was delivered. Alison had two happy years at the Annexe. It was staffed by kind and competent people who taught the students skills that would be helpful to them as they entered adulthood. However, the course only delayed the longer- term problem.

Towards the end of the two years, Martin contacted the then Humberside Social Services Department and arranged for the Director to come and talk to us and other parents; this time questions were allowed. The Director was very honest and open, but had no ready-made solution for Alison and her friends. At the end of the meeting, we suggested that interested parents should meet privately and discuss possible ways forward. So in May 1985 we had the first meeting to discuss going it alone. Through Mary's efforts, this led to us obtaining from the Methodist Church a rent-free building suitable for a sheltered workshop. With plenty of fundraising from all concerned, the Charterhouse Association for Sheltered Employment (CASE) opened its door on 23rd September 1985. (We kept Charterhouse in the name with the intention of giving a sense of continuity to future students coming to us from the Charterhouse Annexe.) Mary was the first voluntary manager and on the first morning six trainees attended – one of whom was Alison. Several dedicated volunteers supervised the activities, which included printing, woodwork, glass engraving and soft crafts. Shortly before the workshop opened, Mary contacted the Humberside Social Services Department to tell them what we were doing. They were surprised that it was all happening so quickly and added £12,000 to the £700 that had been raised over the summer. Apparently the Department had a Voluntary Sector Fund from which this award was made. (The full story of CASE warrants its own place in history.) Two years after opening, CASE moved to much bigger premises at 60 Charles Street, Hull. Over thirty years later, after many changes and improvements, CASE currently supports 140 trainees and employs thirty paid staff. The founding of CASE was another event that had an immeasurable beneficial effect on the life of Alison and many others, both trainees and staff.

As far as Alison was concerned, CASE was work. She attended daily and took her activities seriously. After all, the things she made were valuable, and were often sold at craft fairs, or directly from the CASE building. Year in, year out, she rotated through the various departments, making friends easily with both staff and trainees. We particularly remember seeing her in the glass engraving department (which included leaded glass work). She was dressed in protective gloves and an apron, and was wearing a large pair of protective goggles. She was concentrating very hard and had an electric soldering iron in her hand. The smoke rose off her work as the solder melted and the flux evaporated. We still have a piece of her leaded glass somewhere in the family. We also have two exquisite pieces of tapestry which she produced. It must have taken hours, and infinite patience, by both Alison and her supervisor, to complete them. We have a photograph of a beaming Alison, standing in the reception area at CASE, proudly holding one of them. We remember calling in at CASE one lunchtime and going into the canteen. It was very noisy, with loud music playing and trainees at the pool table, shouting at each other. Alison was sitting in a corner with a newspaper: you could hardly see her behind the opened pages. She was shouting out snippets of news to anyone who happened to be passing by. Latterly, when she worked at the CASE allotments, CASE won the Council prize for the best kept allotment in the City. Alison attended the reception at the City Hall where the awards were presented. When it was CASE's turn to go up and receive their certificate from the Lord Mayor, who was a lady with a stature slightly shorter than Alison, Alison took centre stage and put her arm firmly round the Lord Mayor, in a chummy sort of way, smiling broadly as the Lord Mayor read out the citation. Alison was always concerned when CASE staff were off ill. She regarded them as her friends, and they treated her with particular kindness and affection. One member of staff, Dave, retired due to a heart problem. A rumour went round that he had died. Alison was so concerned that she rang him up to find out if it was true. She did this out of sincere concern, and we trust that she was very diplomatic when Dave answered the phone. No doubt she was pleased to tell everyone at CASE that he was alive and well.

She used to go shopping in town after lunch. She visited lots of shops, buying CDs, DVDs, greetings cards and presents. She got to know the shopkeepers well. Her favourite shop was Ryman's, a national chain of stationers. She was a frequent customer and the staff greeted her as an old friend.

After she had passed away, we learned that she used to call at a particular sweet shop and buy a Twirl (a brand of chocolate bar). As she asked for it, she used to do a twirl to illustrate her request. The shopkeeper said that they always looked forward to Alison calling and brightening their day. She even called in at her dentist, which was near CASE, often to buy toothpaste, but sometimes just for a chat with the receptionists. They told us that she brightened their day too.

In 1987, when Alison was twenty-one, we put on a party for her at a local hotel. Lots of friends from CASE came. Friends from the early years in Wakefield came over as well. We had dancing, games and a supper. The only presents she wanted were a box of chocolates and tickets for an Everton football match. She had supported Everton ever since we moved from Scotland to live in Annandale Road. At the time, we attended the Methodist Church in Willerby. One of the first members of the congregation that Alison made friends with was Mike Britton. Alison learnt from Mike that his father was Cliff Britton, who had spent many years as the manager of Everton. Alison liked Mike very much and, because of this connection, she became a lifelong Everton supporter. With the help of a very good friend of ours, whose father lived in the Wirral and was also a lifelong Everton supporter, we managed to get tickets to see them play West Ham at Goodison Park. Happily Everton won, although the language in the home stand was rather fruity. At one point, Alison turned round to give a supporter in the row behind a hard stare, then turned to Mary and said in a loud voice, "That man swore!", to which he replied, "Sorry love". Shortly after, we heard him shout "Ref, ref, you, you Coffee Pot!"

Alison used CASE to develop her social life. She had several boyfriends and was always faithful to them. At her 21st birthday party she and Steven were an item, and they remained good friends until Steven's unexpected death in 2007. Alison used to telephone Steven every day when she got home, even if she had seen him at CASE. Steven's father worked from home and found long telephone calls in the day a bit of a nuisance, so he asked Alison to leave it until 6 p.m. before ringing. He told us that you could set your clock by Alison's 6 p.m. call. She was very shocked and upset by Steven's death and used to cry whenever something brought Steven to mind. On another occasion, two of Alison's friends at CASE were chosen to represent England at an international football tournament in Geneva. Alison wanted to support them, so we flew over. Alison spent the weekend making new friends, as was her custom, and got herself a weekend boyfriend – a lovely young West Indian man called Arthur. We have a photograph of Alison beaming away with her hand round the neck of a slightly startled Arthur.

During the 1990s, a youth club for young people with learning difficulties was started by a couple of families at the nearby Derringham Bank Methodist Church. Alison attended for about two years before it closed. Whilst there, she had two memorable trips. The first was a trip to Belgium. She stayed on a campsite, sharing our continental tent with other members of the party. Unfortunately, a gale got up and wrecked it, so they had to abandon the site and take refuge in a local flat owned by a friend of the organisers. The second trip was more fruitful. The club went to Morecambe where they all walked across the Bay at low tide. On the way home, Alison phoned us from a service area on the M62. She was clearly excited when she told us of her success and was always very proud of this achievement.

When CASE first moved to its present building in 1987, Alison was living at 238 West Ella Road. Each morning she caught the regular service bus outside the house and liked to sit in a particular seat. This was not usually a difficulty, as the bus was near the start of its route and was normally practically empty. However, there must have been a problem on one occasion, as we found out when Alison arrived home with a large cardboard sign with the words 'Alison's Seat' written on it in bold letters. We think someone must have sat in her usual place and she had probably 'tactfully' said something to the driver, or the passenger (or possibly both!). Whatever had happened, the driver had found a neat way of maintaining harmony on his bus. Alison clearly made an impression on him, as a card and a box of chocolates were left on her seat on her next birthday.

She got a lot of pleasure out of buying presents and cards for others on special occasions. She would buy flowers and a card for Mary on Mother's Day and her birthday. She would buy a very large card for Andrew on Father's Day and a more modest one, usually appropriate and amusing, on his birthday. She had an uncanny knack of buying appropriate cards for particular individuals. At Christmas, she bought calendars for her brothers. She would write all the family birthdays on them, including her own, before wrapping them up and posting them off. She once gave Andrew a diary wrapped in cellophane in a presentation box. He unwrapped the present carefully, opened the diary, and flicked through the pages, only to notice that the page for 2nd November had "Alison's birthday" written in it. Quite how she had got the diary out, had written in it, and had put it back again, without visibly disturbing the cellophane, remains a mystery.

In 1990, we got a real insight into how Alison viewed herself. A mum we knew from West Ella Church had had a Down's baby. Because of family connections, she decided to have the baby christened in the chapel at the Charterhouse Alms Houses (just opposite the Charterhouse Annexe where, five years earlier, Alison had completed her course at Hull College). We were invited to attend and Alison listened to the service without comment. At the end she surprised us by commenting, "She looks a bit like me". We were astonished that she had made a connection with the facial features of such a young baby. Some years earlier, we had been disturbed by an incident that gave an indication of what Alison used to have to put up with. We were sitting round the dining room table, discussing dogs, when someone referred to a particular dog as being a mongrel. Alison straightened up immediately and reacted with clear surprise. It was obvious that the word 'mongol' had, at some time, been used in her presence. Up to then she had hardly been out of the home without us, except for going to school, and we were at a loss as to how she had picked up such a negative term.

We don't know exactly when Alison learnt to swim. After her early experience in the pool at Mudeford, when she was a baby, she saw lots of people swimming in pools during our family holidays. She frequently took to the water herself, equipped with an inflatable life vest. We assume that, on one holiday, the life vest slowly deflated and, without anyone noticing, she just swam on unaided. She also learned to dive off the side of the pool. She became a very good swimmer and took part in many competitions, both at the annual Rotary Disability Games and other organised events. She was awarded several certificates of achievement for different levels of competence. She always had fun in the water and one of her favourite activities was teaching Dad to swim. Being of short stature and with relatively short limbs, by using her superior leverage, she could apply forces he was powerless to resist. She used to teach him by turning him on his back before commanding him to swim. If he didn't obey instantly, he would get a good ducking. There was one particularly memorable incident in the early 1980s, in the outdoor pool at Chamonix, when she decided to give Andrew a surprise. She was standing on the poolside and he was in the pool with his back to her. She took off, landed on his back, and accidently sank her front teeth into the bald crown of his head. Blood was everywhere as he shot off to the shower. His footprints were clearly visible, framed in blood, where he had gone down the steps to the changing room. Eventually, the First Aid department put a large plaster, in the form of a cross, over the wound. Alison's teeth seemed to escape undamaged – she was a tough little cookie. Later on in the holiday, after a few days in the sun, Mary took the plaster off Andrew's head to reveal a well-defined white cross etched on his skull.

One Christmas we bought Alison her first electronic keyboard. It was very small and came with a book of simple tunes and stick-on letters to identify each key. She quickly learnt to read a note in the tune book and play the appropriate key. She was soon playing recognisable tunes, albeit with one hand. Eventually, the stickers wore away, but we didn't need to replace them, because she had memorised the position of each note. We also had a large upright piano and Alison noticed that the pattern of keys was similar to that on her keyboard. We know this because, one day, she surprised us by getting up from her keyboard, going over to the piano, and playing a few bars from one of her tunes. Later we bought her a small piano, and she bought herself a more modern keyboard when she moved into her own flat.

Alison was an avid watcher of professional wrestling on the television. She knew all the wrestlers' names: Giant Haystack, The Undertaker, Hulk Hogan, André the Giant, and others popular at the time. In the early 1990s, Andrew took her to the old Wembley Stadium to watch the World Wrestling Federation's Summer Rumble. The ring was in the middle of the pitch and the rest of the pitch had been covered in what looked like giant pieces of jigsaw puzzle, all locked together. Chairs had been attached to brackets on the pieces and also locked together in rows. They took their seats to watch the first of 14 bouts, fought one after the other, without any intervals. At the start of the evening, the fans were sitting on the chairs; soon they were standing on the chairs; finally, Alison, Andrew, and all the other fans on their row were standing on the backs of the chairs, arms locked together to keep their balance, as they roared their heads off in support of the combatants. Alison played a full and boisterous part in the proceedings. The event was recorded, and we bought the video. On one shot, Alison is clearly visible, standing on the back of her chair, arms linked, and cheering with the others. She watched herself so many times that this particular part of the tape became visibly worn. Unfortunately, when videos gave way to DVDs, the tape was lost.

She gave horse riding a try and joined a branch of Riding for the Disabled (RDA). It operated from stables down a lane behind some houses in East Park (a public park in Hull). She rode regularly, generally at a walking pace, and was fine until she had a fall. After this, she preferred to lead the horses. Prior to the fall, she took part in an RDA regional gala in Wetherby. Les Dawson, the famous TV comedian, was there as the Gala's celebrity personality. He looked lost, standing on his own, not knowing how to react to the disabled youngsters. Alison sorted him out: she went up to him and said, "It's Les Dawson. It really is Les Dawson!" He replied, "Yes it is, love" and gave her a big kiss. After that he was relaxed, and became a different person when interacting with the other disabled riders.

Alison had a knack of speaking quite naturally to the famous. She got a cheery 'Hello' from Buzz Aldrin (the second man on the moon) at a book signing, as she called to him from across the shop. She got another, rather startled one, from an unsuspecting Terry Waite (perhaps the most famous hostage of all time) when she gave him a confident 'Hello Terry' as he walked past us after getting off a cruise ship in Sydney. On a visit to see Thomas in Cambridge, we stopped for coffee at The Haycock on the A1 near Peterborough. Alison said to Mary, "There's Clive Hornby over there" (Clive Hornby played Jack Sugden in the soap opera, Emmerdale Farm). We told her not to be silly, but she insisted it was him. As we were leaving and walking past his table, she suddenly leant towards him and gave him a cheery wave right in his face saying, "Hello Clive". We suspect he had overheard the earlier conversation, because he responded with a big smile, and gave her an equally cheery "Hello!".

One well-known person she saw a lot of was Mark Hill, an internationally famous hairdresser, who has a salon in our neighbouring village of Kirk Ella. Mark always cut Alison's hair personally and was lovely with her. He would even send out for orange juice when she turned down an offer of a cup of coffee. The last time she went to Mark's salon, she spoke to the other ladies waiting for their appointments. She initiated the conversation by saying, "I've got a new boyfriend". The ladies, who had been sitting quietly, immediately pricked up their ears. One of them asked what his name was. Alison replied confidently, "Karl". "Oh that's a nice name," said the lady, to a general murmur of approval. With that, Mark appeared and took Alison round the corner into the salon.

"Now then darling, how are you today?" asked Mark.

"Fine," came the reply. "I've got a new boyfriend."

"Have you darling?" continued Mark, "What's his name?". "Gerard," replied Alison, again with confidence. This response greatly amused the ladies whom she had first spoken to and who could clearly hear her reply. Alison had decided, on the spur of the moment, that Mark, being an important celebrity, would be more impressed by a posh name. After Alison's death a neighbour of ours, who also has her hair done by Mark, told us that Alison was always a breath of fresh air at the salon.

Andrew's cousin, Eileen, was married with four children. They lived in Leicester. The children took up Judo, and the family used to come with the three younger children to stay with us when they were involved in competitions in Hull. Alison used to go along to the competitions as part of the support team. She would get quite excited as each bout proceeded, and was the first to congratulate Eileen's children on a good fight, whether or not they had won. On one occasion, when Eileen's daughter, Andrea, won a cup, to tease her, one of the judges grabbed it and hid it in his Judo jacket. Alison saw this and shot straight across the mat. She confronted the judge with, "What do you think you are doing?". Then, in the full view of the spectators, she plunged her hands inside his tunic and, with one swift movement, retrieved the cup, to the applause of the assembled crowd. Alison got to know her cousins (once removed) very well, and they got to know and love her.

Many years later we received an invitation to the eldest daughter, Eleanor's, 40th birthday party. By this time Eleanor was married and living near Sellafield. Her party was to be held at a hotel in St. Bees. We motored over and, as the hotel came into view, Alison asked us how many stars it had. We didn't know, but the hotel was fine and even had croissants on the breakfast menu: a 'must' for Alison. The party was to be held on the evening of Cup Final day, so in the afternoon we settled in the bar to watch Manchester United play Arsenal in the most important football match of the year. St. Bees is not very far north of Manchester, and the bar was full of United supporters, all dressed in the Manchester United strip. Alison had always had a sneaky admiration for Arsenal, in spite of being an Everton supporter. We watched with increasing interest as Manchester United laid siege to the Arsenal goal, but failed to get the ball in the net. This situation continued throughout extra time, with many near misses, accompanied by groans from the assembled supporters. The penalty shootout to decide the winner proceeded with even scores until the fifth kick, when the Manchester United player put the ball over the bar. At this point, Alison leapt to her feet, punched the air, and let out a great cheer. We didn't know where to hide, as a sea of solemn, angry faces, some in tears, turned to stare at the interlopers. After Arsenal had buried the last ball into the back of the net and won a famous victory, a man sidled up to Alison, put his arm round her, and confessed that he too was an Arsenal supporter, but hadn't the guts to do what she had done.

We kept in touch with Eleanor. One year, she and her family called to see us on their way to catch a North Sea ferry, which was due to sail from Hull. They were going over to the continent for their annual holiday. We were all sitting in a café in Hull's Old Town, when the children started telling 'knock-knock' jokes. Alison decided that she would tell one of her jokes, so she asked, "What is black and white and slides off the table?". Eleanor's husband said, "I don't know, Alison. What is black and white and slides off the table?". Alison replied, "Notts County!". (Notts County is a football team in Nottingham that plays in a black and white strip.) This was not only an unexpected joke, but it particularly amused Eleanor, who had grown up in Leicester, a city practically next door to Nottingham, so had many friends who were Notts County supporters. She promised to use the joke on them.

Alison was a good strong walker and particularly enjoyed walking dogs. In fact, dogs were her favourite animals. At different times, she had two of her own, both West Highland White Terriers. She happily took on the task of training and looking after them with her usual dedication and enthusiasm. Training was largely a case of telling them off when they misbehaved. The first dog, Jessie, had a gentle nature and Alison responded appropriately. When Jessie died Eleanor gave Alison her dog, Scottie. Eleanor's family had bred and shown West Highland White terriers for many years. Scottie was a show champion but had, unfortunately, knocked a tooth out and permanently bent his tail, so he wasn't suitable for showing any longer. He was very feisty and always wanted to be 'top dog'. Alison now owned a dog with 'attitude'. It didn't take long for Scottie to accept her as his mistress, but he was still quite a handful when out walking; however, she managed to control him with her firm, direct and even forceful commands. Alison showed an interest in all dogs and became very good at recognising the different breeds. She startled one woman out walking her dog when she informed everyone in ear shot that it was a Sealyham. When she went for an interview for a placement at a local boarding kennels, she more or less got the job when she saw the owner's dog and told her that it was a Weimaraner.

Apart from domestic pets, Alison liked to feed the birds that came into the garden. She would watch them through a large pair of binoculars. She also used the binoculars for other purposes. Our bedroom overlooks West Ella Hall, a large private house standing in its own grounds. One day she was caught coming out of our bedroom with the binoculars round her neck. She knew that spying on others was not polite so, to avoid awkward questions, she immediately offered the explanation that she had been checking security at the Hall! Some time later, Mary tried to use the binoculars to do some bird watching herself, but couldn't get them to focus properly. We had a look and found that someone (Alison) had unscrewed one of the lenses right out of its housing and then screwed it back in with the threads crossed, so that each lens pointed in a slightly different direction!

When it came to parties, particularly at home, Alison used to give full rein to her considerable social skills. New Year's Eve would see her joining in all the games. When we played Stations, and it was her turn in the middle, she would shout, "All change!" and giggle like mad as the guests rushed around trying to secure a seat to avoid being in the middle themselves. She hosted her own birthday parties, making lists of guests, and deciding on food. When we had charity garden parties, she would do her usual public relations job, going round talking to everyone as she sold raffle tickets; she was a real party girl.

Whilst her brothers were still at home, if Andrew took issue with them over something he was not happy about, Alison would defend them. She would open the sitting room door and say to Andrew sternly, "Into my office". Much to their relief, this threat usually eased the situation. When they left home, she continued to take a keen interest in their progress, and enjoyed all their successes, just as if they were her successes. She told everyone that she had two brothers. We remember when Thomas was getting his degree at Cambridge and was talking to one of his tutors, Alison followed the conversation and, to the surprise of the tutor, chipped in with her own comments. When we went to Sydney to see Giles after he had been away for over a year, she saw him coming down the road and greeted him with, "Hi, Giles!" as if he had never been away. She felt her brothers' closeness and affection, even when they were far off, and she was always very proud of them.

In 1986, Giles started his degree at Imperial College. Alison and Thomas used to come with us to see him, first at his placement in Essex, then at the College in South Kensington. After visiting him in his room at College, Alison would happily accompany us on a walk round Hyde Park, where she once took a photograph of the Serpentine which subsequently won a prize in an open photography competition at Hull City Hall. After the walk and a visit to Speakers' Corner, we used to have a late lunch or early tea at the nearby Cumberland Hotel, which often lasted a couple of hours. Alison loved spending time with Giles and Thomas, and thoroughly enjoyed every aspect of these visits. We, for our part, were quite unaware that we had anyone disabled with us.

Just after Giles graduated, Thomas started his university career at Corpus Christi College, Cambridge. Excursions to see Thomas took the same form as those to see Giles. Visits to Thomas's room were followed by walks in Cambridge and then a meal. On these occasions, Alison got to know some of Thomas's fellow students. They accepted her without the least hesitation and she accepted them quite naturally. Again, we were unaware there was anything special about our family. After his graduation, Thomas moved to London, and our visits to his lodgings picked up where they had left off in Cambridge. During some of these visits, we would stay overnight in a Hilton Hotel. We also stayed in Hiltons on occasional excursions to Scotland. Alison became familiar with what to expect from a Hilton and got used to their four-star standard. She always had a room to herself, usually a double. When she arrived in her room, she had a regular routine: she would put on the TV, do her unpacking, pull back the duvet, put her nightclothes under her pillow, sort out how the shower worked, and finally call us to say that she was 'ready'. We would then go together to find the bar and have a (soft) drink.

In 1999 Thomas married Rachel, whom he had met at College. The wedding was held in a hotel near Rachel's mother's home in Ribblesdale. At the ceremony, Alison confidently read 'The Owl and the Pussycat' to the assembled guests. None of us managed to attend Giles' wedding to Sara in Sydney on 2nd November 2001, but Alison was over the moon when she learned that they had chosen to get married on her birthday.

In December 1992, a 'Crisis at Christmas' hostel opened in Roper Street, a back street close to the centre of Hull. Andrew soon got involved as a trustee and, as he had a small lorry, was asked to pick up donated furniture. Each year the hostel opened at the beginning of December and closed immediately after Easter, when the well-used soft furnishings were taken to the tip. Fresh furniture was needed every year, so each November the hostel advertised on Radio Humberside for unwanted beds, chairs etc. As offers came in, Andrew would receive a fax at work giving him a list of the pick-ups for that evening. After tea at home, Alison and he would pore over a street map marking the various addresses. Andrew would then telephone the first pick-up and arrange to call about half an hour later. They would travel in the lorry to the first appointment and Alison would knock on the door. The occupants, seeing her, had no fear about letting her and her dad in. Her first question would be, "Can we borrow your phone please?". Before loading the lorry with the donated goods, and often whilst Alison was sitting on a settee in the front room, watching a soap opera and sometimes drinking a glass of orange juice, a call would be made to the next address to say that they would be there shortly. At the end of the evening, having visited all the addresses and collected all the furniture, they would go down to the hostel and unload. Alison got to know the hostel staff well. We often visited them, and she made friends with many of the residents too. She always received a warm welcome. When the hostel received a Lottery grant to fit the building out for year-round residency, the nature of the operation changed completely and it became difficult to manage. Andrew resigned as a trustee in the late 1990s and the hostel closed a few months later.

Alison had a very full life when she lived at 238 West Ella Road, but she went on to greater things, as you will see in Chapter 4.

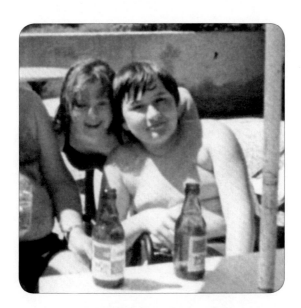

With Thomas in Spain – 1981

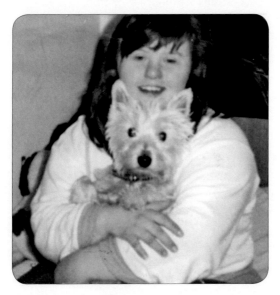

With Jessie 1982

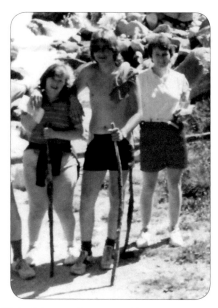

With Giles and Mum – Chamonix 1984

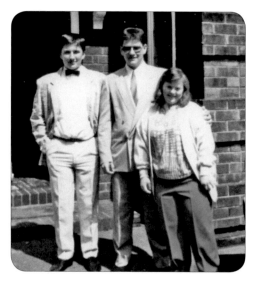

238 West Ella Road – 1986

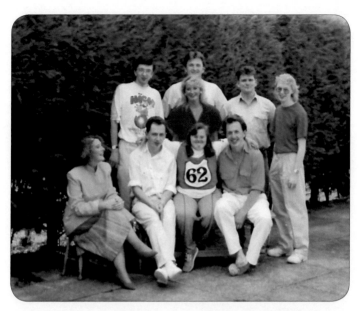

With her Brothers and some Cousins 1989

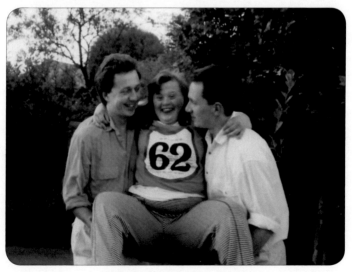

With Nick and Chris 1989

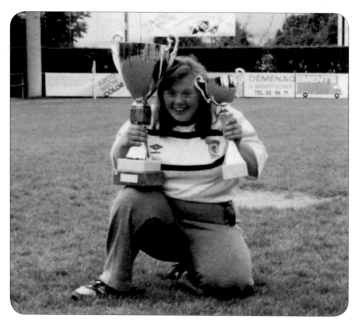

In Geneva with the Football Trophies – 1990

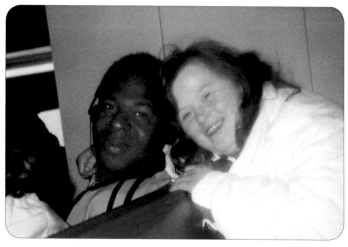

With Arthur (weekend boyfriend) – Geneva 1990

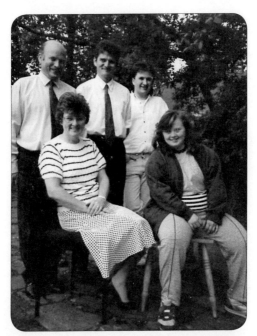

Mum and Dad's Silver Wedding – 1990

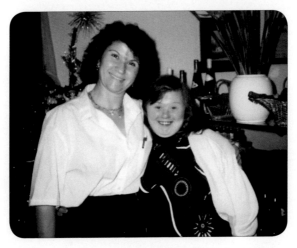

With Bernie (waitress) Jardin Del Sol – 1990

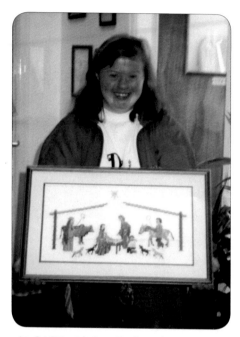

At CASE with her Embroidery – 1991

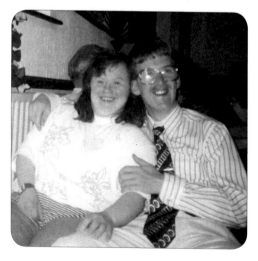

With Stephen (boyfriend) 1993

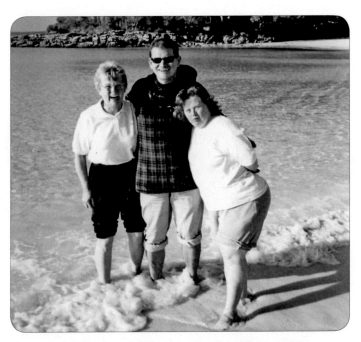

With Mum and Giles at Jervis Bay NSW – 2001

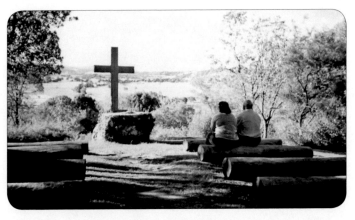

With Dad at Bexhill Open Air Cathedral, Lismore NSW – 2000

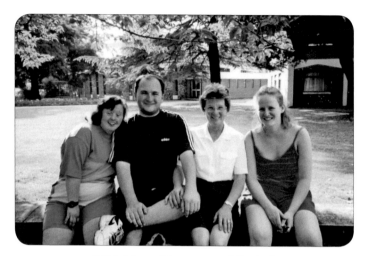

With Mum, Thomas and Rachel

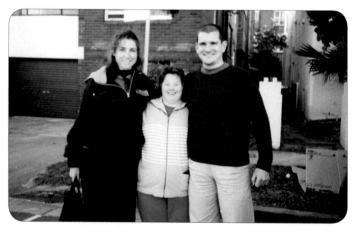

With Giles and Sara – May 2004

Chapter 3

Family Holidays

By our count, Alison visited a total of sixteen different countries. Between Alison being seven and twelve years old, we spent family holidays in Brittany and the Dordogne, first camping and later caravanning. We used to travel from home to our destination without stopping overnight. Alison was the only one to stay awake for the whole of the journey. Andrew would doze off in the queue at Dover and, when the cars waiting to board the ferry started to move, Alison would wake him up with a sharp slap on the head. Red eyed, she would prop herself up in the back of the car between the front seats, keeping a watchful eye on Dad until we arrived at our destination. Once there, she would keel over and fall fast asleep. When we visited hypermarkets she would disappear, only to join us again clutching a tin of pâté (she had an uncanny ability to locate pâté. We've even seen her open a tin without the aid of a key!). She loved camping and caravanning in France: collecting a bucket of ice when the ice van called in the morning; playing boules; visiting cafés and the beach; and sightseeing. We well remember one incident in Pornic, when we were looking for a cake for Giles' birthday. We came across a small shop full of luscious pastries. Just inside the door was a huge gateau sitting on a round display table. None of us actually went into the shop except Alison; she couldn't resist it. She nipped in and, with one quick movement, stuck her finger in the middle of the cake and withdrew it covered in cream and pastry. She had a sublime expression on her face as she sucked her finger. Fortunately, the shop was empty. We made sure we didn't pass it again and set off for the Dordogne the next morning. After five years of camping and caravanning, mainly in the west of France, we decided to venture further south. This meant selling the caravan and returning to camping.

The first place we visited was Annecy, where we camped on the shore of the lake and swam every day. We had a lot of rain in the evenings and at night so, after a few days, we moved south to the Mediterranean and camped on a site at Sainte Maxime near St. Tropez. On our last night the mistral got up. Alison called us at about 4.00 a.m. to tell us that the tent was falling in. We told her not to be silly and to go back to sleep. However, she persisted, so we went through to her compartment. She said, "It really is falling in", as she pushed back the bent corner pole. She was right, it was falling in, so we all got up and were on our way home several hours earlier than we had planned. We had had a great holiday and went back the following year, staying at the same campsites.

After holidaying in the south of France, we went a little further and stayed at an almost perfect campsite near Calella de Palafrugell in north-east Spain. We knew that our GP, Johnny, and his family were holidaying in the same area, so it was not entirely unexpected when they appeared on the site. Soon after they arrived, Alison developed a sore throat, probably as a result of swimming in the busy pool. Johnny got to hear about this and was soon striding across the site, heading towards our tent, stethoscope round his neck. He quickly got the problem sorted. Alison must have been one of very few people to have had her own GP on holiday with her! Johnny is quite a linguist so we were not surprised, when we joined them for lunch in a local café, to find ourselves sharing a table with holidaymakers from all over Europe. Towards the end of the meal, everyone started giving toasts in their own language: "Prost!", "Santé!", "L'Chaim!" etc. Alison watched all this as they went round the table and when it came to her turn she stood up, raised her glass, and said "Up Yours". (She meant "Bottoms Up".) Apart from the amusement it caused, it was a remarkable display of her ability to grasp a situation and respond appropriately with confidence. Since Alison's passing, we have attended Johnny's and Lillian's fiftieth wedding anniversary. After the usual toasts, we all stood and raised our glasses to Johnny's toast of "Up Yours".

In 1984, after another two years camping in Spain, we decided to have a change from camping and beaches, so we rented a chalet at Argentière in the Chamonix valley. For the following few years, we holidayed in and around that area. We used to send post cards to our friends, as you did on holiday. Once, when at a post box, we were confronted by two slots, one marked 'France' and the other 'Foreign'. "Foreign!", said Alison, with great indignation, when she saw Mary put the cards in the 'Foreign' slot. She continued, in the same highly indignant voice, "We're not foreign, they're foreign!". Alison was always a bit diffident about going on the ski lifts which, in Chamonix, were used in summer to reach the high-level footpaths. However, she was very brave and managed well. Once, much to our surprise, she came very slowly down the 'Luge' (a concrete bobsleigh run used in summer, the 'bob' being a sledge on wheels with a simple braking system). We had a final trip to Chamonix in 1988, by which time Alison's brothers were spending their holidays with their own friends. We stayed in a flat on the second floor of a rather dark and sinister looking house which we christened '1313 Mockingbird Hill' (the home of the Munsters, a fantasy family of monsters in an American sitcom). Alison didn't like this accommodation at all. We found this out when we returned from a walk on the first evening to discover all the cases re-packed and lined up in the hall. At the end of the holiday, Alison took a photograph of Dad locking the flat door for the last time. When it was developed, the only thing on it was a close-up of his hand as he turned the key in the lock.

By 1989 Andrew's work situation made summer holidays difficult, so we started to holiday at Christmas. The first year we used the apartment of his brother, Tony, which was near Los Gigantes in Tenerife. For the following two years we stayed at the nearby Hotel Tamaimo Tropical. Alison had always had a habit of drawing our attention to anyone resembling a celebrity. She knew they weren't the actual people, but would refer to them by their celebrity name every time we saw them. The Tamaimo Tropical Hotel proved fertile ground for her 'celebrities'. On the first morning, she quickly pointed out 'Blakey', the ticket inspector from the TV series

'On the Buses'. He certainly had Blakey's depressing appearance and shuffled as he walked. A little later, when we were having breakfast, she whispered, "There's Eric Sykes at the next table": right again, Alison! Later, we had a conversation with 'Hulk Hogan' of wrestling fame. This ability to connect people to celebrities was not confined to hotels. Once, at an airport, she whispered, "The Golightlys have turned up". Mum, Dad and two daughters, all very large, to put it mildly, were walking across the concourse trailing equally oversized cases (the television 'Golightlys', also a very large family, frequently featured on 'You've been Framed', a programme where they performed 'Bull in a China Shop' activities, entering small shops and 'accidentally' knocking over the display cabinets of unsuspecting proprietors). Alison kept this amusing habit up over many years, and latterly referred to Mary's friends from the village, Audrey and Kate, as Audrey Hepburn and Kate Winslet.

It was on one of these holidays that we heard Alison knocking on something in the middle of the night. It turned out that her slatted bed had fallen apart and she was putting it back together. She remembered this experience and, whenever she encountered a strange bed, she would lift the mattress and have a peep at the base, just to make sure it was sound.

We used to hire a car to drive round Tenerife. We visited the usual tourist attractions: Mount Teide, the Drago Tree and, of course, Loro Parque. One Christmas, we went into a church near the Drago Tree. Inside was a full-size stable, on a stage, in front of the Altar. Inside the stable was a crib, complete with a life-size ceramic baby Jesus. Two children, a boy and a girl, both about eight, were the only other people there. When they saw Alison, the boy motioned her to come forward onto the stage. She stood at one side, looking a little uncertain, as he crept quietly up to the crib. He gently lifted out baby Jesus and took him over to her to hold. She held the baby, cuddling him for a minute or two as if he was real. She then gave him back to the boy. He crept back to the crib, all the time making a shush sign with one finger on his lips, before he kissed baby Jesus gently on the forehead and laid him down. Then, smiling at Alison, the two children ran out of the church. It was a lovely scene acted out by all three of them with great reverence.

We often ate out on these Christmas holidays and tended to revisit the same restaurants time and again. Alison soon got to know the various waiters and waitresses, and they remembered her from year to year. We were dining at one of these restaurants late on the evening of 5th January. The following day was Epiphany when, by tradition, presents were given to children. The restaurant was called the 'Jardin del Sol', and the waitress, Bernie, had hit it off with Alison from our very first visit. During the evening, she told us that the Three Wise Men would be arriving in the local square to give out presents. Mary shot off to get one for Alison from a nearby shop and took it straight to the organisers. Just after midnight, we went to the square to welcome the Wise Men, who arrived on horseback, beautifully clothed and wearing turbans. Alison scrambled with all the children to pick up sweets scattered by the men; then she watched the children receive their gifts. She had no idea that there was one for her, and reacted with alacrity when she heard the name Alison Peeech called out. She confidently ran forward to get her present, and was really excited to be part of the celebrations as the onlookers cheered and clapped her.

In 1991 Andrew's elder brother, Mike, retired and went to live in Portugal so the focus of our holidays switched to the Algarve. Alison loved to visit Mike, who lived in a bungalow out in the hills, in an area called Eiras Altas. He had several aviaries where he kept brightly coloured finches and other exotic birds. He also had a Labrador dog called Meg. Alison loved feeding the birds, walking the dog, and considered sweeping the terraces her personal responsibility. By the time we made what turned out to be our last visit to see Mike, in late 2002, Alison was living independently in her flat on Kingston Road and did not come with us. It was at the end of October, the time when we put the clocks back on the Saturday night. Her watch, like all digital watches, was tricky to change. However, we had a friend, Malcolm, lined up to help. We phoned Alison on the Sunday morning and, although she was fine, something in the conversation did not quite add up. Mary asked her what time it was. She gave Mary a time two hours later than it should have been. Malcolm had altered her watch the wrong way. Apparently, a quick call from Alison brought him hurrying back; as Alison put it, "He hadn't even had a shave". She solved this problem for future occasions by keeping two watches, one set to Greenwich Mean Time and the other to British Summer Time: a typical Alison solution.

Alison had many short holidays at Aldeburgh in Suffolk. We had been going there with Aunty Chris and her family for Easter breaks since the early '80s. Alison threw herself into these visits and got to know the area well. Aldeburgh has an inshore lifeboat and one day, when it was out on exercises, she joined the semi-circle of spectators who had gathered to watch it come ashore. As it beached and the crew climbed out, with much applause from the crowd, Alison stepped forward and shook hands with each crew member and congratulated them. The crew were completely at ease, responding naturally and kindly to her gesture. The last time we went to Suffolk was in April 2014. We visited The Red House, at one time the home of Benjamin Britten and now a museum dedicated to his life and work. It was closed for refurbishment. Seeing Alison's disappointment, the caretaker let us into the garden, and even gave us a fork to dig up any vegetables we would like to take. So Alison, having visited Suffolk regularly for 30 years, spent part of her last visit helping herself to Benjamin Britten's vegetables. She was always very respectful of those who had passed away, and knew, from a previous visit, that Benjamin Britten was buried in the church cemetery at Aldeburgh. Later that day, at her request, we took her to the cemetery, where she watered the flowers on his and Peter Pears' graves. At the end of the holiday, we asked her what had been the best part; she replied, "Digging the vegetables".

In the mid-to-late 1990s we spent a week on a very long narrowboat. We did the Stourport Ring. Starting in Bromsgrove we went down the River Severn to Worcester, then up various canals, passing by Cadbury's factory at Bournville and Gas Works Basin in Birmingham, before making our way back to Bromsgrove. Alison was a bit unsure getting on the vessel but, once established in the forward saloon, she happily read the canal maps and offered relevant bits of information as we chugged from lock to lock. She got quite used to the rocking motion, which she took in her stride, and to getting off and on the narrowboat at points of interest. Our friends Peter and Delia, Delia's sister Beryl and her husband Ken, were part of the team. Peter was an experienced sailor with a steady hand at the tiller, but Ken was not so skilled, particularly when navigating some of the tight tunnels on the route. He had a habit of knapping off the odd brick that was protruding from the lining, thus covering the roof of the barge with brick dust. The noise, when he did this, was quite startling. Alison would be at the front of the boat, watching where we were going, and Andrew would be at the back, ready to push the boat off the side of the tunnel. Whenever we heard the clatter as Ken hit a brick, Alison would stand up, glare down the length of the boat, and shout accusingly, "Dad!". In fact, it didn't matter what went wrong, the call would go up, "Dad!". On that holiday, to show her appreciation, Alison bought gifts for everyone. Having left Beryl and Ken on the boat, we went to a book shop where she made her purchases. As she was choosing a book for Beryl, who had very poor eyesight, Delia commented, "Beryl can't read", to which Alison replied with disdain, "Well she can learn!".

We had another holiday with Peter and Delia, this time in Devon, at the home of Peter's elderly uncle Bob who was a retired vet. Alison loved Uncle Bob and, when the time came to leave, her comment was, "I'm staying here with Uncle Bob".

At Christmas 1997 we holidayed in Orlando, Florida. The weather was so poor that the water parks were closed. This didn't deter Alison one iota. We saw all the shows in Disneyland: 'The Little Mermaid'; 'The Hunchback of Notre Dame'; and, on New Year's Eve, a fantastic production of 'A Christmas Carol'. We visited the MGM Studios, The Epcot Centre, Sea World and the Space Centre at Cape Canaveral. She enjoyed every minute of the holiday but, at Cape Canaveral, refused to go inside the rather realistic mock-up of a Space Shuttle. On the flight back, a child in the seat behind Alison annoyed her by continuously kicking the back of her seat. Suddenly, the child's mother started hitting Alison on the head and saying, "Excuse me, excuse me, what do you think you are doing?". It transpired that Alison had somehow managed to force her hand between the seat backs and flapped the child's tray up and down a few times. The lady was not pleased, but the child was quieter after that. Subsequently, we twice took Alison to Disneyland Paris. She took up where she had left off in Florida, and particularly enjoyed trips on the small train that ran round the perimeter of the theme park.

In March the following year, Andrew sold his business. Therefore, we became free to take holidays at any time, not just at Christmas, so we had a week in Madeira in late autumn. The hotel had a minibus to take residents down to the centre of Funchal. Alison would climb onto the bus and sit next to the driver, as if by right. This amused the driver and the other passengers, who were mainly German, and they soon cottoned on and made sure she got the front seat. Alison, of course, knew they were German from the language they were speaking. The first time we were in the hotel lift with German guests, out of the corner of her mouth, and in her stage whisper, she said to Mary, "Don't mention Hitler". On another occasion, early one morning, when Mary and Alison were going down in the lift dressed in their swimming costumes, ready for a dip before breakfast, one German lady asked, "Are you going to the pool?". Before Mary could stop her, Alison replied, "Yes, we are going to get there before the Germans". She had obviously absorbed the stereotypical German habit of putting towels on sunbeds.

She had her birthday whilst we were there. To celebrate the occasion, the hotel brought a birthday cake to our table. It was far too big for us to eat so, after Alison had blown out the candles and we had each cut ourselves a slice, we asked the staff to cut the rest up and offer it to the other guests. The British guests gave us a wave from their tables and mouthed a polite 'thank you' but, without exception, every German who took a piece got up, came across to our table and gave Alison a kiss saying, "Now we can enjoy your cake".

By this time, Giles had moved to Sydney and in May 2000, Alison made her first journey to Australia. When she saw Giles it was from the balcony of our apartment at Coogee. He was walking up the road towards us. She was the first to see him and greeted him from above with her usual "Hi Giles", as if he had never been away. During our stay, Giles took us to the Homebush Olympic Park, the site of the 2000 Games. It was just a month or two before the opening ceremony, so everything was ready. We had taken with us 'Barney Bear', a toy from a primary school close to West Ella. We had been asked to do a 'Barney goes on Holiday' feature for the pupils. Alison took Barney onto the main track, placed him on the finishing line, and took a photo for the feature album.

We toured all the venues and finished with a swim in the pool at the Aquatics Centre. Later on we travelled by car to Mullumbimby to meet some friends of our future daughter-in-law, Sara. On the way we stayed at Byron Bay, a town famous for hippies and whale watching. Alison was very keen to see a whale, so much so that the proprietor of the B & B, who had warmed to her as soon as we arrived, lent her some 'far-lookers' (the word some Australians use for binoculars). He told her that she was guaranteed to see a whale as he had painted one on each lens. She did in fact see several whales from the local lighthouse.

After Alison had charmed our new friends in Mullumbimby, we set off back to Sydney using a scenic route. We stopped at a wayside café, where we met a family with a Down's daughter about Alison's age. The daughter took Alison off to show her their caravan whilst we had coffee with her parents. They told us that there was a very effective early intervention programme in Australia for children with Down's. After the girls had returned, we said goodbye to the family and set off again. Leaving the main road, we took a scenic route towards Wiseman's Ferry. Eventually the road came to a chain-driven ferry taking cars across a lake into the town. Alison wanted to stop and buy some sweets and a film for her camera. We also needed some petrol. Andrew and Alison went to a petrol station for the fuel and sweets, whilst Mary went to another shop for the film. Alison rifled through the shop shelves looking for marshmallows. Having found some and paid for them, she then went back to the car. As Mary returned, she met the man from the petrol station coming out of the shop crying. It transpired that his wife had given birth to a Down's baby four weeks earlier. The family were of Pakistani origin and had been given very little information, other than that their daughter would be unable to do very much for herself. He had never seen an adult with Down's and was surprised and emotionally affected when he saw how 'normal' Alison was. Mary told him what Alison could do and how she could read and write. Alison showed the man her holiday diary and he asked for a page to show to his wife. We told him that Alison didn't want to spoil her diary, but would write his wife a message. On a blank sheet of paper torn from her diary, and with Mary bending over so that Alison could use her back as a rest, Alison wrote, "My name is Alison Peach. Don't worry about your new baby, she will be a little cracker". Mary then went on to tell the man about the early intervention programme. We left him still in tears.

Alison went back to Australia with us the following year. We stayed with Giles and Sara in their rented house in Beaconsfield Road, Chatswood, North Sydney. The house had an outdoor swimming pool which Alison made full use of. It also had cockroaches and a resident Huntsman spider, none of which thrilled her. During her two stays in Sydney, she enjoyed all the usual tourist activities: going to the Opera House; crossing on Sydney Ferries to Manly Beach and Darling Harbour; and regularly watching the buskers whilst sitting in a café at Circular Quay. Probably her favourite attraction was Sydney Aquarium. She also saw 'Annie' live on stage. She bought the video and played it at every opportunity. We took a river trip to Parramatta. Once there, we went into a café for a cool drink. Andrew ordered a passion fruit dispensed from a large, transparent container which was sitting on the counter. It had a paddle which constantly rotated, stirring up the freshly squeezed fruit. Little black seeds were swirling about near the bottom of the tank and Alison, with her usual sangfroid, confided to Mary, "He won't like it. It's got flies in it."

Unfortunately, on the flight home via Seoul in South Korea we had exceptionally bad turbulence over a long period. Alison had always been nervous of flying and when we got home she said that she would never fly again: she was as good as her word.

Alison had stopped flying by the time Thomas and his family first went to live in Australia, but when his company moved him back to Amsterdam in 2007, she came with us to visit him on several occasions. She knew her nieces well, as they had stayed with us in West Ella for some weeks, before finding permanent accommodation in the Dutch capital. On visits to see them, she fitted almost seamlessly into their new life. Mary recalls one tender moment when Alison got up from the dining table, taking a banana with her, and sat on the floor to eat it. Jessie (then about two) immediately got down from the table taking her yogurt with her, went over to Alison, sat down on the floor close up to her, and started eating it.

When in Amsterdam, Alison used to walk with Katie to her new school. She also walked with Alex to her kindergarten and with all of them to the local swing park. When Rachel took the children to the larger Vondelpark on her box bike, she would walk with us to meet them. Alison used to love visiting the museums in Amsterdam and would wander off on her own, looking carefully at the various Van Gogh and Vermeer paintings. We also took her, at her request, to Anne Frank's House where she joined the Anne Frank Society.

Trips to Amsterdam entailed long car journeys via the Channel Tunnel. One was undertaken in very thick snow and we had to stay overnight in Kent, due to the motorway being blocked. We were lucky to get two rooms but no food was available except dry bread rolls, which we had for both supper and breakfast. We were on the road for 36 hours and, apart from being amused, Alison took the whole episode in her stride. Just once, we went by North Sea Ferries. It was a large vessel but it still rocked, and Alison was extremely afraid throughout the whole of the crossing.

After Andrew retired, we all joined the David Lloyd Sports Club at Kingswood, in North Hull. Sue and Colin, whom we had known for many years, joined about the same time and we used to play tennis with them. Alison would often come with us to watch, after which we would all go for a swim in the pool. Colin was a fierce competitor and occasionally fell over in his efforts to return the ball. On one occasion he hurt his back, and was clearly in some pain. Alison witnessed this. From then on, every time we met, she would look at Colin, hold out her left hand, rotate it backwards and forwards with her little finger and thumb extended, and ask, with an impish grin, "Any twinges, Colin?". We became very friendly with Sue and Colin and used to visit them in France, after they had gone to live close to the Pyrenees. They lived in a very old stone farmhouse, part of which was thought to have dated from Roman times. Sue and Colin named one of the bedrooms 'Alison's Room' which, naturally, she used when we stayed. They also had an apartment in Alicante, which we all thought Alison would enjoy visiting. Sue and Colin asked her if she would like to have a holiday there. She beamed as she said "Yes", and only looked a little askance when we explained that it would mean a plane flight. However, she still said she would "give it a go". She came with us to book flights for a week's stay at the end of October.

A few days after we had booked for Alicante, and the day before we were due to travel to France for a holiday with Sue and Colin, Colin fell off a ladder while pruning a tree and broke his pelvis. By the time we arrived, he had been hospitalised in nearby Argen. We all went to see him. We found him laid flat on a hospital bed with various coloured ropes threaded through or round parts of his lower body. One rope was keeping a leg up in the air at an angle of 45°. He was clearly in considerable pain. Nevertheless, Alison went round the bed, bent over him with her face close to his, and demanded, "You will be alright for Spain, won't you, Colin?"

Later that holiday, Sue took her Peugeot to a garage for servicing and Alison went with her. Alison liked travelling in Sue's car because it had a hood that let down. We followed in our car and, later in the day, took them back to collect Sue's car. Sue settled up with 'Gerard', the young man behind the counter. On leaving, Sue shook his hand and gave him a peck on each cheek. Alison watched this with interest, and then offered her hand to Gerard, which he took. With a vice like grip, she slowly pulled Gerard over the counter, and down to her level, before planting a full-lipped kiss firmly on his cheek. She looked very pleased as we left.

When the day finally arrived for us to fly from Manchester Airport to Alicante, Sue and Colin were back in Hull. We had involved Alison in every aspect of the trip, in an attempt to get her to 'take ownership' of the flight. We all set off together, although Alison was a little quiet. At the airport, we handed in our baggage and went through customs. Then we all went to a restaurant to get some breakfast. We sensed that Alison had a growing apprehension, but we were all taken aback when the flight was called, and she got up in floods of tears, and hid behind a pillar. Mary immediately went to the flight desk to warn the staff that they might have to get the cases off. The chief stewardess came to try to persuade Alison to board, but to no avail. The pilot came and invited her to go and see his 'office', but again, to no avail. We finally waved goodbye to Sue and Colin as they walked down the tunnel to board the plane. The airline staff were excellent; they were very sympathetic and had already off-loaded our luggage. We were shown out of the airport by a back door, and we went straight to a café to work out what we were going to do next.

We were determined to have a holiday because we thought Alison, just like everyone else, needed one. We set off for Wales with mainly euros for currency and beach clothes in our cases. After stopping to kit ourselves out with warm clothes, we finally booked into a B&B just outside Aberystwyth. All in all, we had a nice few days in Wales, before stopping off on the way back at Holmfirth. This is where one of Alison's favourite TV programmes, 'Last of the Summer Wine', was filmed. We had tea in the café where Compo, Clegg and Foggy used to meet, and then we took a tour of the various film locations in a bus similar to the one used on the sets. We paid our respects to Bill Owen (who played Compo) in the town cemetery, where his memorial includes a pair of wellingtons. We were pleased we decided to have this holiday because Alison, as always, took a keen interest in everything we did and particularly enjoyed the visit to Holmfirth.

Using the Internet, Alison discovered that her great-grandfather's brother is commemorated on a panel at Menin Gate. She also discovered that her grandmother's cousin was killed in the First World War whilst flying over the lines in northern France, and is buried in the Warlingcourt Halte Cemetery. We went over to France and took her to the cemetery to see the grave. She went straight to it, having taken with her a plan of the cemetery, which she had previously printed off from the Commonwealth War Graves Commission website. We took her to Ypres, where we attended the daily service of commemoration at Menin Gate. It was a Sunday evening and a full service was held. It was attended by representatives of many local military units. Alison watched silently as they marched, in full uniform, from the town's market place to the Gate. She was in the congregation as The Last Post was sounded and flags were lowered. It was very emotional. We also visited many other war cemeteries with her. Some were small groups of gravestones in isolated villages next to swing parks; others were more extensive. Alison took a respectful interest in everything connected with the fallen.

We first met some of our dearest friends, Claire, Thibaud, and their three daughters, when Thibaud, who is a heart specialist in Paris, had been seconded to a research project at Castle Hill Hospital in Cottingham. His family came over with him and lived in the nearby village of North Ferriby. When they went back to Paris, we kept in close touch, and they often came to stay with us when Thibaud returned to Castle Hill to follow up his project. On one of his return trips, Alison told Thibaud about her family tree and showed him photos of Menin Gate. He told her that his grandfather had died in the First World War. Alison carefully noted the name and, when he returned a few months later, she produced a photo of a grave. Thibaud was astonished and asked, "How did she get that? That's my grandfather's grave!" Later we all went over to Paris for a few days, and stayed with Claire, Thibaud and their daughters at their home in Bourg-la-Reine. We had a delightful time, and Claire, Thibaud and the girls were excellent hosts. They were most particular to make sure that Alison was included in their family life. Claire came over for Alison's funeral and the family sent us a lovely card of condolence. They recalled that when we stayed with them we had visited Parc de Sceaux, a nearby country house popular for weddings. Being a Saturday, there were lots of brides having their photos taken in the grounds. Alison did her fair share of congratulating and, we suspect, got on one or two of the pictures.

We look back over our holidays with Alison, and count ourselves extremely fortunate to have been able to share so many adventures and experiences with her.

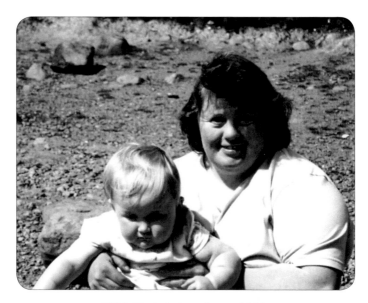

With Katie in London - 2002

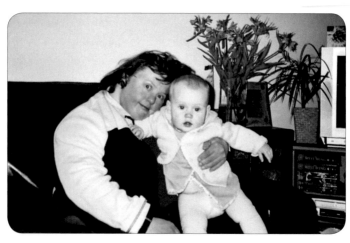

With Alex in London - 2004

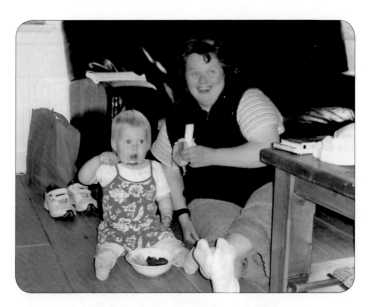

With Jessie in Amserdam – 2008

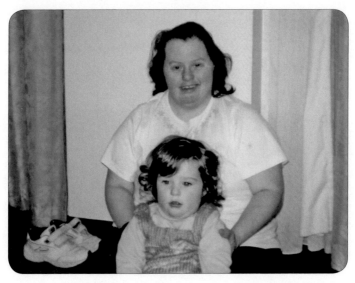

With Moira in England – Christmas 2008

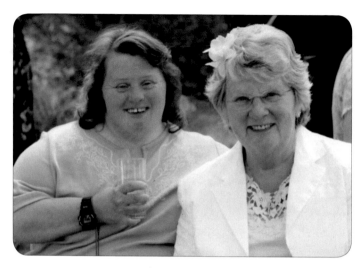

With Mum – 2007

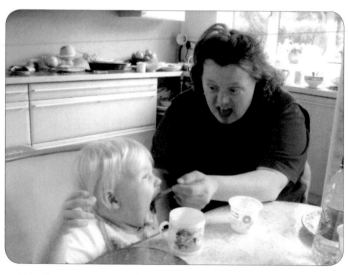

Feeding Jessie – Kitchen at 238 West Ella Road – 2007

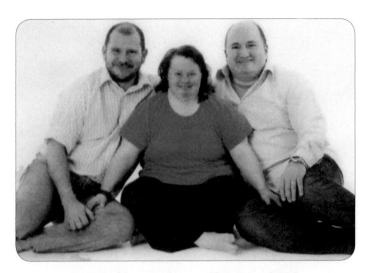

Proud of her Brothers – Christmas 2008

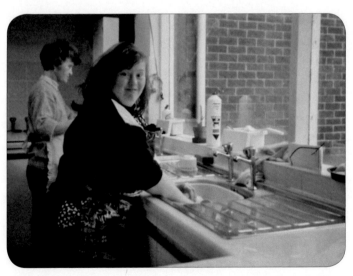

Washing up at Leisure Day – Willerby Methodist Church

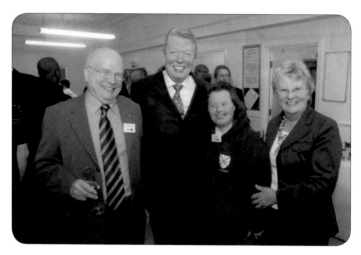

With Alan Johnson (former Home Sec.) –
Case 25th Anniversary

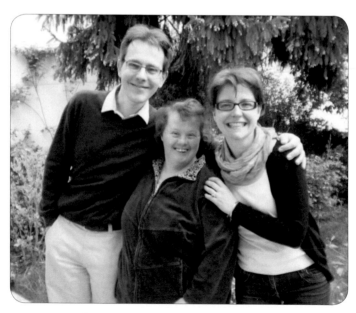

With Claire and Thibaud in Paris – 2011

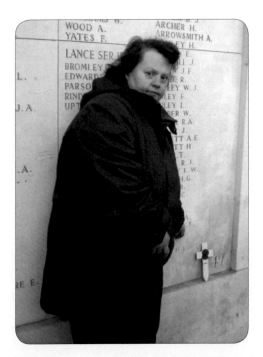

Remembering a Great Great Uncle - Menin Gate, Ypres - 2011

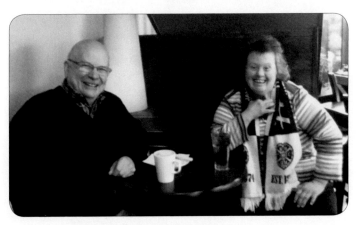

Back in Hull at Planet Coffee with Dad

Chapter 4

Alison in her own Flat

In 2001, Alison had a boyfriend called John whom she met at CASE. He lived in his own flat where occasionally she would go for her tea. We think this prompted her to announce, out of the blue, that she would like her own place. It was an unexpected request, because we had been considering downsizing for some time but if we even looked at a 'For Sale' board in her presence she would say, "We're not moving!". We decided to strike whilst the iron was hot so we set about finding her a flat. As luck would have it, one came up to rent less than two miles from where we live. It was a furnished, two bedroomed, ground floor apartment at 167 Kingston Road, Willerby. Situated on the corner of Kingston Road and the Parkway, it was one of only two flats in the building, the other being on the floor above. The sitting room picture window overlooked a busy roundabout; shops and a pub were nearby, and there were frequent buses to Hull. We took Alison to see it. As soon as she got over the threshold she said, "I'll have it". She moved in on 19th March 2001. In May 2002 Alison's landlord decided to sell the property, so she was able to buy her lease with the help of her own mortgage. When we told her that she now owned her own place, she said, "Great", followed by, "Dad, can I have some more paper for my computer please?". Alison getting her own flat was another event that had an immeasurable effect on the quality of her life and her self-esteem.

She made very good friends with her neighbours, who all admired her for living independently. They were also surprised, you could say thrilled, by the way she regarded them as equals, and interacted with them accordingly. The first couple of times we went to Australia without her, she simply stayed in her flat and looked after herself until Aunty Chris arrived and, effectively, substituted for us. Throughout the time we were away Alison carried on with her usual daily routines, although we believe Chris spoiled her quite a lot. On the third occasion we went to Australia without her, Aunty Chris invited her to go and stay in Stourbridge. Before going, Alison confided to her neighbour, "I'm being shipped off to Mum's sister's, you know".

Alison was well known to her local shopkeepers. She used most shops on a regular basis. On her first Christmas, she put a Christmas card through every shop door. One of the shops had been converted to a French restaurant and was run by a local celebrity called François. He could often be seen standing at the restaurant door, and when Alison passed, she would hail him with "Bonsoir François", and he would reply (no matter what time of day or night it was) "Bonsoir, Alison". At the time that Alison took up residence on Kingston Road, another CASE trainee was living nearby. She was called Sonja and used to get on the bus a couple of stops after Alison. Other trainees also caught the bus nearer town so, by the time they got off, there was a small group of young people with her as she walked from the bus stop to CASE; the sequence was reversed on the way home. Alison and Sonja soon became good friends. Twice a week, Sonja would stay on the bus as far as Alison's stop, where they would get off together, walk to Alison's flat and have tea. Sonja lived at her parents' pub in Aston Road. Alison often went there by way of a change, and was loved and respected by Sonja's parents and siblings. As a treat, on dark Friday evenings in winter, we would pick them both up from CASE, and take them straight to Alison's flat. In the car it was like being a fly on the wall, as we heard them discussing who was going out with whom, and listened to any accompanying scandal. Sonja remained a good friend and still came to tea until a few months before Alison died; however, by this time Alison was back living with us.

Bearing in mind that Down's are the most watched people in the world, we knew exactly why Alison was so fond of her flat. When she got home, she would take off her coat, go into the sitting room, kick off her shoes, sit in her chair, put her feet up, and switch on the television: no one was watching; no one was interfering. With her bedroom and sitting room doors open, she could see the television from her bed, and found that she could put on or turn off the TV using the remote without getting up. She always liked to have music on when she was not watching TV. She had a karaoke machine which would take three CDs. She would set this going when she went to bed, and go to sleep to the music. She particularly liked David Soul songs: in fact, using the Internet, she did a project on him, part of which we still have. At the beginning of the project she wrote, "David Soul has plenty of children". What a sweet way of describing his family, and so typical of Alison!

She used to do her own cooking and cleaning. She did her main shopping with us at the weekends, but always insisted on having her own trolley. She made her own choices and paid with her own money. She liked croissants with soft cheese for breakfast. She often made sandwiches which she took to CASE for lunch and, in the evening, would cook a pre-prepared meal in the microwave when she got home. The only hot drink she liked was Oxo, and she usually drank flavoured waters. At first, we used to ask her if the meal was cooked right through, to which she would reply, "It's piping hot", just to reassure us that it was more than adequately heated. Curiously, in other circumstances, she would use the expression 'stone cold' if something was not warm enough. At the weekends, she would come to us for her main meals, but after eating, unless there was something special happening, she would ask to go home.

The regularity with which she washed her clothes took a toll on her washing machine. She got to know 'Dan the Washer Man' quite well. One day her machine stopped working completely. Dan, who was a big man, framed the kitchen door, looked at her sternly as she was standing next to the lifeless machine, and said, "You've wrecked it." Alison's face was a picture of contrition, until she saw him give her a wink. The gas engineer who used to service her boiler recalled that she gave him 'a hell of a grilling' on his first visit. When she answered the door to his knock, he said, "I've come to service your boiler." He told us her response was, "No!", and she shut the door in his face with a heavy 'clunk!' He checked that he had the right address, and then tried again but got the same result: "No!" Clunk! Earlier, we had received a call from the engineer to say that he was on his way to Alison's, so Mary was already going there to meet him. Mary arrived just in time to sort things out. But, as the man said, he should have had some identification on him to show Alison and, without it, she was quite within her rights to refuse him entry.

Alison had had her own current and deposit accounts with Santander even before she moved into her own place. The bank had a branch at the Willerby Shopping Centre, about half a mile out of Willerby. On moving to Kingston Road, she transferred her current account to the Willerby Post Office, which was nearer and more convenient for her to use. Later she moved her current account to the NatWest bank in Willerby Square. She would draw out the same amount every week and would hand the cashier a list of the notes and coinage she required. She did this so that she could take the right money to CASE for lunches, pay the correct amount for her weekly contribution towards her TV licence, and have enough notes for her weekly shop, with some left over for spending money. It became apparent that it would be better to transfer her savings account (still at Santander) into her current account at NatWest, so that everything was in one place. We went to Santander with her to make the change. We had all the necessary documentation. Nevertheless, the young man behind the counter found it extraordinarily difficult to understand what Alison wanted to do. Eventually he excused himself, got off his seat, and went through the door behind him into the back office. As he did so, Alison turned and asked, "Is he thick or something?". Eventually, we got the transfer done.

As her first Christmas in her own flat approached, she told us that we would be having our Christmas dinner with her. When we attempted to suggest otherwise, she firmly informed us that we had to go because she had already bought the paper plates. On the day, Mary helped with the cooking and we had a lovely time together.

She used to keep in close touch with us using both her landline and her mobile. She would use her mobile to phone us in the morning when she was on the bus going to CASE, and again when she got home at night. Once, late at night, when she had been to the pictures in Hull with her then boyfriend, John, she called us from the back of the bus station to say John had left her and caught his bus home; we quickly went and picked her up. On another less serious occasion, early one morning we got a call from her when she was still in bed. She said, "Dad, there are two little animals playing on my bedside table". We assume they were ants, which had disappeared by the time Andrew arrived.

On a weekend early in 2002, we went to London to see Thomas and Rachel. They were expecting their first child and we had gone to do some last minute decorating before baby arrived. Alison stayed in her flat and, unbeknown to us, had asked her boyfriend, John, to stay overnight. At about midnight, the phone rang in Thomas's house: it was Alison. "Mum, can you come round straightaway, John is having a fit." We knew that John suffered from epilepsy and it transpired that she had already called John's brother, who had then called his Dad. Whilst we were on the phone, his Dad arrived at the flat at the same time as an ambulance and the police. It was a bad epileptic fit and John, after emergency injections, was taken to hospital and kept in for some days. Mary managed to speak to John's father and asked him to make sure Alison was O.K. before he left her on her own. She coped with the situation admirably. If she hadn't raised the alarm, who knows what the outcome might have been? When we came home a couple of days later, empty syringes were still lying on the bedroom floor where the medics had thrown them after injecting John. Referring to this episode in later years, Alison would say, "I saved John's life you know," and she may well have been right.

On another occasion she was waiting with a friend at the bus stop for a bus to take them to CASE. Without warning, the young man had an epileptic fit. Alison knew what was happening and what to do. In fact, she appeared to be the only one at the bus stop who knew what to do. As the bus arrived, she was kneeling beside him, holding his head on one side and keeping it off the pavement. The driver phoned for an ambulance and all the passengers got on the bus and left Alison, with her friend still on the ground, to wait for the ambulance. When it had been and gone, she phoned us to tell us what had happened and to say that she had missed her bus. We shot down to the stop, only to find that she had already caught the next bus to town.

Whilst she was at CASE, Alison had three long-term placements. The first was at Lowna Kennels, at nearby Raywell. She started there whilst still living in West Ella and attended one day a week for 15 years. She helped with bathing and grooming the dogs, washing food bowls, cleaning kennels, looking after cats, and general fetching and carrying. She was popular with the staff, who were mainly teenage girls. She liked cats and they seemed to like her. They instinctively recognised her as a friend, and even the most timid would go to her for a stroke, or to sit on her knee. She left this placement because she felt she needed a change. Her new placement was at 'Home from Home', another boarding kennels. These kennels were in Swanland, a village quite nearby. At this placement, the owners went out of their way to praise her for her genuinely useful contribution to their business. In the 1990s, Alison took a part-time course in general animal management at Bishop Burton College. We attended the College Open Days with her and she was always greeted warmly by the College staff.

At the same time as she was working at 'Home from Home', she had a placement at Willerby Methodist Church, which was less than half a mile from where she lived. Thursday was the Church's Leisure Day, and Alison went every week between the beginning of October and the following Easter. Her main job was to help to serve lunch to about eighty old people. She wrapped the cutlery in paper napkins, served the puddings and washed up afterwards. She used to walk home when she had finished, and then do her own housekeeping. She used to give us a call as soon as she got home to let us know that she was back. She was popular with the staff there too, and they always invited her to their annual Christmas outing, usually a meal in a restaurant. Because of this placement she was well known to many local pensioners, who would greet her warmly when they met her when out shopping. Often, after an encounter with an elderly lady, Alison would confide, "She's one of ours", meaning of course, that the lady was a 'customer' at Leisure Day.

In 1985, one of Alison's friends, Cath, from the West Ella Methodist Church, decided to move with her husband and family back to her home city of Edinburgh. Unbeknown to us, Alison wrote to Cath asking her not to move and telling her how much she would miss her. It was a well written, properly addressed and dated letter. We only found out about it when Cath gave us a copy of the letter after Alison's funeral.

Some years later, Alison started to travel to Edinburgh and stay with Cath and her husband, Armando, for a few days each year. We would put Alison on the train at York and off she would go to Waverley Station, where Cath and Armando would meet her. We had lots of 'fun' getting Alison seated on the train at York. The problem was that the train only stopped for a minute or so and we didn't have time to get Alison and her luggage on, settle her in the correct seat, and get off again, before the train left. Our first attempt at solving this problem involved Mary having a word with a lady member of staff who happened to be on the platform: she promised to help. A few minutes later she came back and said that she was sorry but she had to load a bicycle. However, her colleague, Brian, (whom she indicated with a wave of the hand) would help. Brian cut an unusual figure, being a very short, stocky individual in a rather large, British Railways peaked cap. The train duly came in. Brian was temporarily engaged with arriving passengers, so Mary got on with Alison. Andrew was standing at the train door trying to catch Brian's eye when, to his horror, Brian waved his flag and blew his whistle to herald the train's departure. Andrew immediately put one foot on the train and left the other on the platform. The driver shut the train doors, or rather tried to, but as they closed, Andrew firmly pushed them open again. After a further three or four unsuccessful attempts by the driver to close the doors, Brian looked round to see what the problem was. He soon realised the cause and came running over. Andrew became aware that Brian was round his knees, with both hands on the train door, trying to hold it open. Suddenly, Mary appeared, having run down the carriage, propelling other passengers in front of her, and jumped smartly off, just as the doors slammed shut. After this episode, we decided to contact the rail Helpline. We were told that the next time Alison was travelling we were to let them know in advance. They would arrange for a staff member to see Alison onto the train; the staff member would be waiting for them at the Station Information kiosk.

The following year, we did as they suggested, and contacted the Helpline a few days before Alison was due to travel. This time, she was catching the 11.00 a.m. train from York and going right through to Glasgow to stay with friends there. 'Fiona', from the kiosk, seemed to get Alison on the train and seated in seconds, so when she got off we asked her if she had put Alison in the right seat. She said, "No, but I'll phone the guard and ask him to move her". After an hour or so, Alison gave us a call on her mobile, as was her custom, to report in. We asked her if she had been moved; she said she hadn't. Later, she phoned and said that she had been moved by the 'Netball girls'. Obviously, the girls had got on, found Alison in one of their seats, and moved her into another carriage. This worried us because we had told our friends in Glasgow which carriage Alison was in, so we phoned them to let them know of the change. Then Alison rang again to say that she couldn't find her coat. We concluded that she had left it behind when she was moved, so we called the Helpline. They were very sympathetic and assured us that they had full details of Alison's journey. They said that they would phone the guard on the train, get him to sort everything out, and then call us back within 15 minutes to confirm everything was in order. After 45 minutes, they called to apologise and say that they had searched the wrong train. They had searched the 11.00 a.m. train from Kings Cross not the 11 a.m. train from York. However, they said their staff at Glasgow would meet the train, find the coat, and make sure Alison was fine. In the event, Alison called to say she had found her coat, and then our friends called to say they had found Alison. As far as we know, the train company staff never showed up.

The next time she went to Edinburgh we had the help of 'Kevin'. On this occasion Alison's boyfriend, John, went with her. We got to York early and met Kevin at the Station Information kiosk. He took us over to platform 13 where the London to Edinburgh train was due to stop. Right on time, a mainline train came thundering in to a neighbouring platform. Kevin immediately told us that the platform must have been changed and that this was the Edinburgh train. We moved quickly across to the new platform and Kevin, with Alison and John right on his heels, got on. Whilst Kevin was seeing them to their seats, a lady came up to Mary and asked her if this was the train to Newcastle. Mary said it was (the Edinburgh train invariably called at Newcastle) and confirmed it by pointing to a notice, clearly displayed on the side of the coach next to the door, saying 'Newcastle'. With that, Kevin got off. Just to be certain, Mary pointed to the notice and asked him to confirm that the train did, indeed, go to Edinburgh. The blood drained from Kevin's face. He shot down the platform waving his arms and shouting "Stop, Stop" at the guard. Kevin had put them on the wrong train. Luckily, he managed to get them off and put them on the correct train which had, meanwhile, pulled into the original platform. After that, Alison travelled First Class. She would be met at the train door, escorted to her seat, her luggage taken care of, and then offered juice and a cake. She always had a big smile on her face as the train pulled out of York station.

In Edinburgh, Alison usually went to watch Heart of Midlothian play football and she became an ardent Hearts fan. As a special treat, on one visit Cath arranged for her to visit the Club on a training day. She met the players and was invited up to the trophy room. The players quickly took to her, and she was photographed with her arms round their star striker, who was much revered by the local fans. She came home with a signed and framed Hearts team shirt and group photo which she hung above her bed in her flat.

She once went on her own by coach to Birmingham, where she was picked up by one of her twin cousins and taken to her Aunty Chris's house in Stourbridge. Looking back, our confidence in her ability to cope with any situation must have been very high. Without any fuss, we just put her and her luggage on the coach and waved her off.

She had another coach holiday, this time on one of the National Coach Company's trips to a hotel in Eastbourne. She went with her boyfriend, John, who had been on similar trips before. Again, we waved them off without too much concern, and picked them up a week later when they got back to Hull. Alison was beaming as usual. When we asked her how she had got on, and what the other holiday-makers had called her, she said, "I'm fine. They called me John's girl."

Music and musicals played a large part in Alison's leisure pursuits. She built up quite a collection of CDs and DVDs. As a special treat, usually once a year, we would take her to London to see a show. We had a special number to call to get theatre seats which were reserved for disabled people. Apart from being half price, they were usually towards the side and near the front of the stalls. The seats had masses of leg room to accommodate wheel-chair users. We took her to see 'Joseph and the Amazing Technicolor Dreamcoat', 'The Lion King', 'The Sound of Music', 'Mamma Mia', 'Billy Elliot', and, lastly, 'The Wizard of Oz' with Michael Crawford playing the Wizard. Towards the end of each show, members of the audience would move to the front and join in the dancing. Alison would be there with them, dancing and singing every word. We often noticed members of the cast making eye contact and winking at her as she gustily sang along with them. Alison naturally took an interest in the Royal Family, and enjoyed a trip to Buckingham Palace, where she saw an exhibition of the Queen's dresses and had tea on the terrace.

When we were out in the car, she would comment on other drivers' motoring habits, particularly when Mary was driving. Sometimes she would mouth comments at offending drivers, which could be quite worrying. Other times, if someone cut in or otherwise misbehaved, she would say in a loud deliberate voice, "I saw that". This would be followed by "Thank you" as she nodded at them when Mary passed them. If any learner driver came into view, Alison would say, "She's failed (or he)", whether or not they were struggling. To entertain anyone who was present, she would make small words out of number plate letters by inserting any necessary additional letters herself. She would also perform small, but sometimes alarming, driving tasks, like pulling on Mary's handbrake when she came to a stop in the drive.

When Alison spent time with us on winter weekends, she and Mary would often bake chocolate buns. Alison would carefully put the icing on with a table knife and then decorate them with tiny white chocolate stars and other coloured shapes. She always put plenty of buns aside to take home.

By the time CASE celebrated its 21st Anniversary, Alan Johnson, the West Hull MP and former Home Secretary, had become a Patron. Alison responded to his affable manner and regarded him as a friend when she met him at CASE. It was quite natural that she, as the only trainee from the initial intake still attending, and Alan, as Patron, should together cut the 21st Anniversary cake and later the 25th Anniversary cake. As well as Alan Johnson, other well-known visitors came to CASE. She met Tommy Steele, one of the early rock and roll stars, whom she later saw at Hull New Theatre when he played Scrooge in the pantomime 'A Christmas Carol'. She met Cathy Staff and Stephen Lewis, both from 'Last of the

Summer Wine'. Stephen also played the part of Blakey in 'On the Buses', the person she had 'spotted' years before, at breakfast, in the hotel in Tenerife.

Alison was never into politics but was aware of the political personalities of the day. When Edwina Currie, the then Secretary of State for Health, announced that eggs were contaminated with salmonella, Alison referred to her as 'the lady who put salmonella in eggs'. Alison always voted Labour after she had seen a Party Political Broadcast in which Neil Kinnock sang a duet with Tracey Ullman (at that time, a pop star).

We made a big effort to make Alison's 40th birthday a special occasion. We took over the lounge at the Hull Ice Arena, put on a disco and a buffet, and hired a chocolate fountain. On arrival, every guest was given a medallion on a lanyard to keep as a memento. It had a picture of a dolphin and the words 'Alison's 40th – I was there' engraved on it. Eighty-five guests attended: many of her friends from CASE, friends she had made from Rotary and Inner Wheel, friends from her work placements, friends from Willerby and West Ella, other friends from over the years, some from Scotland, families from as far south as Berkshire and as far north as Cumbria, as well as Giles from Australia. Thomas would have liked to be there but needed to stay with Rachel who was awaiting the birth of their third child. It was a splendid occasion and, at the end, everyone joined hands in a circle and sang CASE's unofficial anthem, 'You'll never walk alone'; there were several tearful eyes from people outside the learning disabled community. The following day, a Sunday, guests who had travelled from afar met for lunch at a restaurant only a couple of doors from Alison's flat. It was another noisy and enjoyable event. Towards the end of the meal, a taxi arrived to take Giles to the station to start his long trip home to Sydney. So ended a celebration which, in its way, was a very fitting tribute to Alison.

We first met Rena and Bobby, who come from Lennoxtown in Scotland, when we were on a cruise celebrating our 40th wedding anniversary: Alison had stayed with Aunty Chris in Stourbridge. We invited them to come to West Ella for a weekend. Alison came to meet them and to join us for a meal. As the time for the meal drew near, Mary asked our guests if they liked the food she was preparing: specifically, she asked if they liked leeks. Bobby said that he wasn't too sure as they had a funny texture, to which Alison, looking straight at him, replied, "Tough". Rena nearly fell off her chair laughing at such a direct but unexpected reply. Later, Bobby told us that he thought Alison was brilliant. We saw them several more times in the following years and, during a visit to Castle Howard, Bobby took a photo of Alison on the café terrace. It was this photograph that was used on the Order of Service at her funeral, and appeared in the Hull Daily Mail tribute to her. Bobby and Rena came down for her funeral and remain our very good friends.

Whilst at CASE, Alison took up with yet another boy, called Adrian. He lived in a monitored flat at Keyingham, a rural village east of Hull. Once, he travelled all the way from Keyingham by bus to see Alison in her flat. He brought his computer tower with him. We don't know what he wanted to show Alison, but he managed to get the tower working using her monitor, keyboard and Internet connection. Later in the year, we dropped her off at one of CASE's regular Friday night discos at the local

Trades and Labour Club. Thomas was staying with us at the time, and he went with Andrew to pick her up. They arrived just in time to see Adrian climb onto the stage, take the microphone, and announce his engagement to Alison. Judging by her reaction, she was as surprised as we were; however, she reacted appropriately as her friends rushed to congratulate her. This relationship finished abruptly after she visited him at his flat and apparently found his intentions a bit too much for her liking.

Alison was keenly interested in her family tree and remembered spending time with her grandparents and other relations of their generation. In fact, shortly after Andrew's mother died, when Alison was only five, a lady with a good resemblance to Andrew's mother passed by in a car. Alison immediately declared "Mamie's back" (Andrew's mother liked to be called Mamie by her grandchildren). By the time Alison was living in her own flat, the use of the Internet made it easy for her to pursue her family history interest. She quickly learned to open ancestry.com and similar sites, fill in names and other details, and search the records. She would print out the results and put them in a file for future reference. As well as relatives killed in the First World War, she discovered children who had died in infancy of whom we knew nothing. She also discovered relatives who had been killed in the Sheffield Blitz: Andrew's family came from Sheffield. She unearthed many addresses where her great grandparents and various aunties and uncles had lived. We treasure her records which we have been careful to keep.

As a follow-up to her research, visits were made to Sheffield where Andrew had real 'daddy and daughter' days exploring the areas his ancestors had lived in over a hundred years earlier. In the early 1900s, Alison's great-grandfather, Byron Peach, had been one of a group of people known as the Sheffield film makers. He had acted in silent movies, as well as filming and developing them, and then projecting them in makeshift cinemas. We knew that he had galloped on horseback through Endcliffe Woods, dressed as a cowboy. We also knew that he chased a crook across the balcony at Sheffield Town Hall dressed as a policeman. We visited both these locations and photographed many houses that her ancestors had lived in, often very close up and with the current occupants visible in them! According to the 1901 census, at the age of 17, Byron had been a potboy in the Red Lion, a pub on London Road where his stepfather was the licensee. We had lunch there, but not until Alison had explained to the current landlord our connection with his premises. On more than one occasion we had lunch at the Woodseats Palace. This is a Wetherspoon pub built on the site of the former Woodseats Palace Picture House, where Byron had been the cinema manager throughout the Second World War, and had finished his working life before retiring to Bridlington. On her first visit, Alison had a word with the staff and was directed to the upper level where there was a photo on the wall of the old Cinema as it was in Byron's day. He and his wife are buried in Bridlington, and Alison used to insist on visiting their grave every time we were in that area. She always took a bottle of water and filled up the birdbath on their grave. We also visited Leeds where she took photos of various flats where her Uncle Michael had lived when he was just starting out on his working life.

From 2000 until 2014, Alison attended the Rotary Disability Games. These games were held every year on a Sunday in April. We used to take a coachfull of competitors from CASE to locations as far apart as Sheffield and Cleethorpes. The Games usually started at 9.00 a.m., so we needed to leave CASE premises by 7.45 a.m. As service buses were not very frequent on a Sunday morning, we arranged for Rotarians and willing parents to pick up competitors from all over Hull, starting at 7.00 a.m. A few weeks before the Games, competition forms were sent to CASE so that each competitor could tell us their address, and record the events they wanted to enter. As the final date for the return of the forms drew near, Alison would collect them and bring them home. She would check the details, then put the appropriate postcode into the computer, and print off a map showing the location of each house. This was preparatory to putting together a list for Rotarians to make the necessary collections. She loved helping with this work, which she realised was important, and it gave her a real sense of achievement. She herself always competed. She entered swimming and two knockout events: Boccia, a sort of soft ball indoor bowls; and New Age Kurling, which uses plastic 'stones' on ball bearings in place of the granite stones used in the normal game of curling. She would accept defeat with her usual good nature, and cheer on her friends, congratulating them and celebrating their success with enthusiasm. She got to know her last boyfriend, Kevin, when he attended the Games for the first time. He was tall, thin and extremely well-mannered. He had an affection for Alison which, initially, only extended to asking after her politely. Later, he was always pleased to see her and greeted her with a warm hug. He remained her faithful friend right up to her death.

Our Rotary and Inner Wheel friends greeted Alison as an equal, and warmly welcomed her at social and fundraising events. Alison would take charge of the washing-up in the café at craft fairs and auctions. At one auction, she took a fancy to a full size pottery Labrador dog with a broken toe. She happened to be sitting at the side of the main hall behind a column which practically obscured her from Ken, the auctioneer, who was a Rotarian she knew well. When the dog came up for auction, she proceeded to bid. It soon became apparent that there was another lady in the audience who was equally determined to get this item. After each bid by the lady, Alison popped her head round the column and raised her hand to increase her bid. Ken was becoming quite concerned as the amount started to go way above the value of the dog. Finally, a woman sitting next to Alison pointed out that the dog had a broken toe, to which Alison replied, "I can live without it", and stopped bidding, much to Ken's relief.

Every December, Mary asks the residents of West Ella to donate items to the Salvation Army's 'Christmas Toy Appeal'. The generosity of the village residents is overwhelming and our home is regularly filled with beautiful presents. The Salvation Army officers used to receive addresses of deserving families from the Social Services Department. Club members would then make up parcels of toys which were appropriate to the ages of the children and deliver them in person. As you can imagine, this activity was right up Alison's street. We well remember taking her to a house on one of the big estates in east Hull. It was dark outside but still early evening. Lights were on, but when we knocked no one answered the door. A glance through the letterbox revealed shoes scattered in the hall, a dog running round, and sound from a television in the sitting room. After a few minutes trying to raise someone, we told Alison that we would make another delivery and then come back. We arrived back about half an hour later only to have the same problem; but this time, the shoes had gone, the dog was nowhere to be seen and the TV had been switched off. Possibly in frustration, Alison lifted the flap on the letterbox and shouted, "Come on, open up, we know you're in there". She never did get to deliver that particular present but had great joy in giving gifts to many other families.

Alison rarely had a health problem; she didn't even need glasses. She was always very strong and physically fit. She used to go off to work in the worst of weathers and hardly ever had a runny nose. Although she knew her doctor, Johnny, very well socially, she didn't like going to see him professionally. We can only remember one occasion, when she had a small cyst that needed removing, that she actually visited the surgery, apart from seeing the nurse for her annual flu jab. We were therefore surprised and totally unprepared for what was to unfold over the next two or three years.

Chapter 5

2012 Onwards

Over the years, the premises occupied by CASE Training Services started to show signs of wear and tear. Grants totalling £1.4 million were obtained in 2012 to refurbish and extend the building. This necessitated vacating the premises for an estimated six months. The building closed in the July and Alison was transferred to Festival House, a building in the pedestrianized part of Jameson Street, where CASE had obtained a short term lease for the first floor. Only the more capable trainees were sent there and she found herself in the company of her more able friends, including Sonja. However, the usual activities ceased and were replaced by deskbound work. Alison managed this change without any problem. The short term lease on Festival House was extended by a further six months, but finally came to an end in July 2013, with the refurbishment of the main building still not finished. Alison's group was split up and each trainee relocated. Alison was separated from her friends and put with a much less able set. Again, the activities bore little resemblance to those Alison had enjoyed prior to

July 2012. Although the staff were good, she hardly knew them, and found this change hard to cope with.

Just after Alison joined this new group, we went to Australia for four weeks, leaving her to stay with Aunty Chris in Stourbridge where she was her usual happy self. Shortly before we went, Alison's cousin, Sue, who worked on the set of the soap opera, 'Emmerdale', invited her to a family day at the studio. It was an occasion when members of the production team could invite their close relations to visit the 'village' and meet the 'stars'. This was perfect for Alison and she had a wonderful day meeting and being photographed with all the celebrities. She had obviously been a 'hit' with them too as, at the end of the visit, the cast asked why she had not been invited before! Shortly after returning from Australia, we went to see Chris to thank her for looking after Alison. We visited a local pub for lunch and bumped into a group of Chris's friends. In conversation with them, Chris mentioned that she had choir practice that evening. One of the ladies asked what she was doing; as quick as a flash Alison, in her 'don't be silly' voice, replied "Singing". Alison was in good form.

However, when she returned and went back to CASE, we got a call saying that she was trying to leave her department early. They thought that she was afraid of missing Sonja, whom she travelled home with, and who was now in another department. By December, her friends at her placement at Leisure Day were concerned because she was becoming less communicative. Something appeared to be undermining her confidence. We had a further illustration of this early in March 2014, when she came with us to meet Giles in London; this involved staying overnight in a hotel. Usually, she was fine in her own room and coped perfectly well without any help, but on this occasion, she could not be persuaded to stay in her room on her own, and Mary had to spend the night with her.

Later that month Alison, along with the other trainees, moved back into the refurbished and extended main building. Not only had the internal layout been totally altered, but none of the old practical activities, except catering and IT, had been retained. The new 'workshops' were more like classrooms and designated Academic 1, Academic 2, Ability 1 and Ability 2. In contrast to the former activities, the new activities were mainly deskbound. There had also been significant staff and organisational changes, with more emphasis being put on welfare, which entailed the welfare department taking a more prominent role with each trainee having a designated welfare officer. Both the staff and the trainees (now called clients) were encouraged to report any 'incidents' to 'welfare'.

By the late autumn, we started receiving evening calls from Alison saying that she "didn't feel too good". These continued with increasing frequency over a period of several weeks, culminating in her telling us that one of the trainees had called her an unpleasant name. She seemed to be unable to put this behind her, and was becoming so upset that we decided to support her by staying with her at her flat overnight: Mary one night, Andrew the next. We managed to sustain this for quite some time on a four-nights-a-week basis: Alison coming to us for Friday, Saturday and Sunday nights. Then we started to sleep badly and, by the spring of 2015, Andrew's health was beginning to be affected so, very reluctantly, in April we moved her back to 238 West Ella Road. It was hoped that this would be a temporary measure whilst we got to the bottom of Alison's problems. We took her to see the doctor and he gave her anti-depressant medication. Later she started to jerk shortly after waking. These jerks could last for an hour or more, so the doctor took her off her medication and told us that the jerks were nothing to worry about.

Alison attended CASE throughout this period but we found it necessary to take her and bring her home by car. At CASE, she was displaying fight or flight symptoms (usually flight) typical of someone suffering from depression. This was very noticeable when she came into contact with the trainee who had called her an unpleasant name. In an attempt to alleviate the situation, we arranged for Alison to spend most of her time at CASE's allotments, where she had several friends amongst the trainees, and liked the staff.

For some time, staff at CASE had been suggesting that Alison should follow the practice of some of the other trainees, and engage a personal assistant to be paid for out of her Personal Budget. This was money she had a legal entitlement to but which had not, at that stage, been given to her by the East Riding Social Services Department. Hence, at the beginning of 2015, she engaged Jenny. Alison had been leading an independent life for many years and saw no need for supervision; however, she was well aware that Jenny was there to keep an eye on her and 'help' her when necessary. In spite of her best efforts, Jenny did not find it easy to engage with Alison, who continued to show the flight side of her reaction to depression.

It must have been a referral by Alison's doctor which led to our first visit from an NHS nurse who specialised in people with learning difficulties. She came three times in all and, after initial suspicions about why the nurse was there, Alison got on well with her. The nurse was amused and surprised by Alison's quip when she suggested that Mum and Dad might need a break: Alison cracked back immediately with "They can have a Kit-Kat". That was the end of that conversation! ('Have a break; have a Kit-Kat' was a well-known phrase used to advertise a popular chocolate bar.)

To maintain her interest and vitality, Alison's Social Services Care Coordinator suggested additional placements. All trainees at CASE had to have a Care Coordinator in order for CASE to receive financial support from the Council; Alison had had one for several years. One placement turned out to be a short spell at a Social Services day centre in Hessle, where she did well and was generally happy. However, she didn't like some of the activities, particularly keep fit and dancing. Nor did she like the level of supervision when they went out as a group, and she tended to want to establish her independence and go off on her own. Social Services were unable to cope with this and her placement was terminated abruptly. Another placement, initially suggested by us, was at Mires Beck Nursery, a garden centre near North Cave. This was founded many years ago, by friends of ours, to support learning disabled people by engaging them in horticultural activities. Alison spent one day a week working with Jenny in Sandra's greenhouse. Sandra was a lovely lady, just right for Alison.

We had been concerned for some time about how Alison would get on after we had passed away. Quite unexpectedly, a place became vacant in a home we had known and visited over several years. This was called Harry Priestley House, a Masonic care home situated about 30 miles from West Ella, in the town of Thorne. We were confident it was as suitable as it possibly could be, bearing in mind that no one, especially Alison, would like going into a home. After several trial nights that appeared to go well, Alison moved in in mid-October 2015. However, within a few days things had become difficult. Perhaps understandably, she was not sleeping at night and was disturbing other residents. This was surprising to the staff, as the long-established residents were very quiet and well behaved. The only shot in the staff's locker to deal with this was medication, which the local surgery was happy to dispense. On the 17th day of her stay, early in the morning, having had five different drugs during her stay, Alison had a seizure in the shower. She was taken to Doncaster Royal Infirmary where she had several further seizures. We stayed in the hospital with her for six days, before she was discharged. We took her back to West Ella and she didn't return to the home. The hospital discharge letter gave the cause of the seizures as 'changes in medication'. On returning to West Ella, we took her to see a specialist who diagnosed apraxia, a brain disorder that affected the ability to move the limbs, to swallow and even to speak. We also learned that the jerks the doctor had dismissed earlier that year were myoclonic jerks and a possible precursor to epilepsy.

Between December 2015, and May 2016, we spent many happy days with Alison, both at home and out and about. However, her ability to control her legs and arms slowly deteriorated and she steadily lost all but a few words of speech. Latterly, she started having difficulty swallowing. In March we had an unsuccessful attempt to get help from an agency via Social Services but were more successful in getting advice from a range of specialist nurses from the NHS. At the beginning of May, Aunty Chris came to stay for a week. At the end of her stay, Chris said she thought that Alison had deteriorated noticeably since she had arrived. Over the next three weeks, with the help of equipment supplied by the NHS, we were able to nurse Alison at home. In her final week, she was seen by both clinicians and nurses, who all failed to spot that she had contracted pneumonia. The day before she died, we had a morning visit from a nurse who was concerned about Alison's inability to swallow. The nurse showed Mary how to thicken Alison's drinks but also said that she thought Alison had a chest infection. By the afternoon, Alison had a strong ruckle. Being Saturday afternoon the doctor's surgery was closed, so we asked Johnny, now partially retired, to call round. He diagnosed advanced bronchial pneumonia. He said it was far too late to do anything except make her comfortable and keep her mouth moist. Our good friend, the Rev. Jonathan Jukes, Vicar of St. Andrew's Church, Kirk Ella, came round straight away and read the 23rd Psalm to Alison. She clearly heard him as, having been asleep in bed and very still, she wriggled and wriggled as he spoke. We knew she was not afraid because she didn't call out as, even then, she would have done if distressed. She then went to sleep for the last time, just waking once at about 10.00 p.m., opening her eyes very wide, and giving her mum a lovely kiss on the lips. She passed away, peacefully and with dignity, in her sleep at just after 7.00 a.m. on the morning of Sunday 29th May 2016.

The courage with which Alison coped with her last few weeks, and her bravery when facing death, is a supreme example we will all struggle to follow. Giles had been over three times in the previous twelve months and spent time with her on each occasion; however, despite leaving Sydney as soon as the situation became clear, he didn't arrive until the day after she died. Thomas had come over and spent a week with Alison. He left the day before we were told of her pneumonia. He got the news of Alison's passing when he was at Dubai airport. He offered to turn round and come straight back, but we felt it was better for him to continue on his journey home and see his family before returning for the funeral.

After Alison died, we had over 400 cards and other messages of sympathy. The Hull Daily Mail printed a full page tribute to her, and a further forty tributes appeared on their Facebook page from people we did not know: some had met her on the bus or at the bus stop; others had served her in shops she used to frequent in town; and still others knew her as a neighbour. Many CASE staff and trainees came to Alison's funeral, and a few weeks later a service for her was held at CASE's premises in Charles Street. Prior to the service, a reception was held in the canteen. All Alison's CASE friends were there. The service was conducted by the Rev. Jonathan Jukes, who had read to Alison the afternoon before she died and had later taken her funeral service. The large upper room at CASE was packed and several emotional tributes were paid to Alison by her friends. A video compilation of photos of Alison at CASE and on CASE outings was shown. One of them was of her in a canoe, well wrapped up and paddling on a very windy lake. We did not know she had ever been near a canoe, and don't know, to this day, how they got her into it! We still see her friends from CASE and they always speak kindly of her.

On the day of her 50th birthday, five months after she had died, we were leaving her flat in the evening, having closed her curtains, just as a small group of ladies was passing by. We caught a snippet of their conversation: they were saying what a nice lady she was and how she always spoke to them when they met her. Mary could not resist asking them if they were talking about Alison. They were, and they went on to speak most kindly about her, and to say how sorry they were to read of her death in the Hull Daily Mail.

Kirk Ella Church was full to overflowing for her funeral, which took place on Friday 10th June. Friends attended from as far away as Scotland and Paris. Both Giles and Thomas came over from Australia and each spoke about their memories during the service. Giles told the assembled congregation that Alison did not choose to have Down's Syndrome, that it was not a career decision or a lifestyle choice but a life which came with considerable hurdles, but Alison had faced them all with a mixture of humour, straight talking, courage and an iron will. He was sure they all had memories of when Alison had exceeded their expectations, challenged their perceptions, or lightened their day; sometimes all at the same time. He said that what she had achieved in her 49 years was extraordinary. Thomas recalled that Alison always knew what she wanted to do and was always ready to fight for it. All her life she had been dealing with the low expectations of people outside the family, and all her life she had been beating them. He said that his children never saw Alison as their disabled Auntie; she was just Auntie Alison. She was the bravest, kindest, most loyal and loving person he had known.

That is the story of Alison Mary Peach, the lessons she taught and the joys she brought. Everyone she touched was a better person for knowing her.

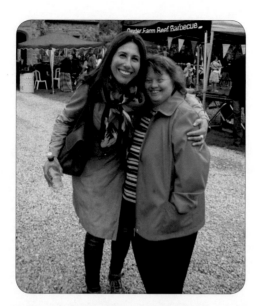

With Gaynor Faye at Emmerdale Studios – 2013

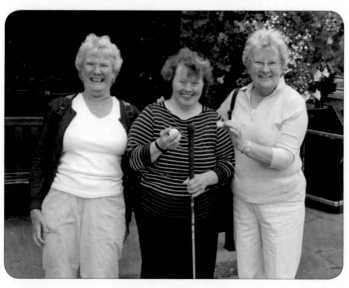

Putting with Mum and Ena at Bridlington – 2013

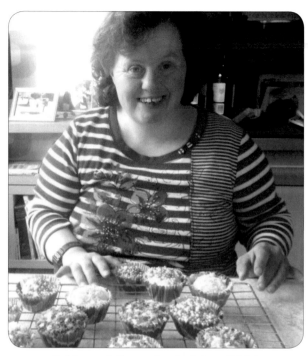

Baking – A Favourite Activity – 2014

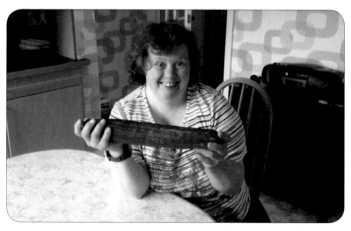

Cucumber – Grown at CASE Allotments – 2014

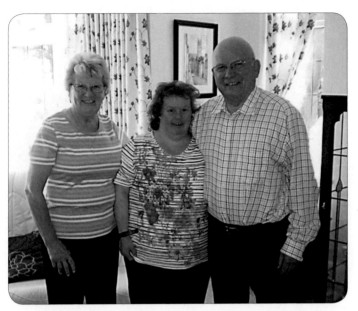

With Mum and Dad at 238 West Ella Road – 2014

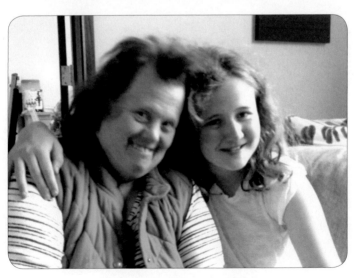

With Katie in Devon – 2015

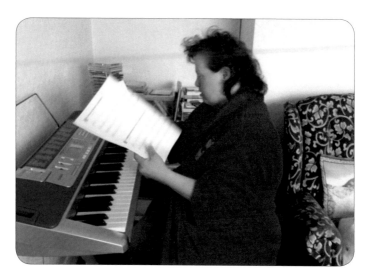

At her Keyboard – 167A Kingston Road – 2014

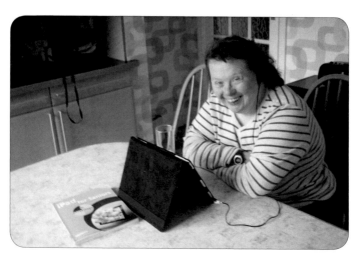

Listening to Music on the iPad – 2014

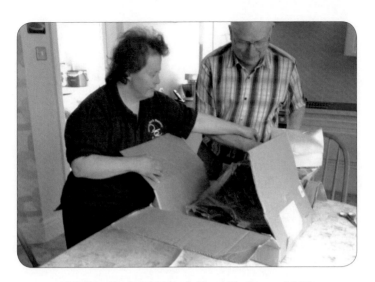

Helping Dad to Unpack New Clothes – 2015

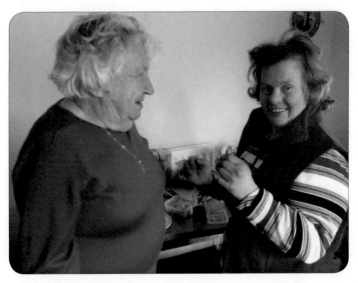

With Aunty Chris at Stourbridge – April 2016

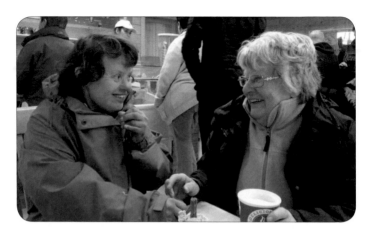

With Mum in a Café at Honeysuckle Farm, Hornsea –
April 2016

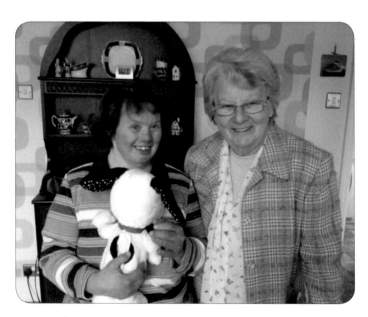

With Mum in the Kitchen at 238 West Ella Road –
April 2016

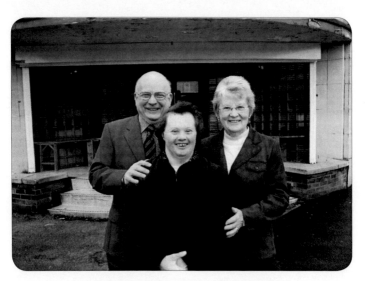

With Mum and Dad outside CASE

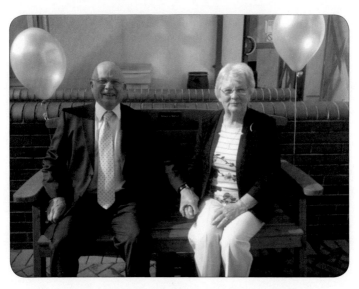

Sitting on Alison's Memorial Bench at CASE